# A MODERN HERBAL

## ALYS FOWLER

MICHAEL JOSEPH
*an imprint of*
PENGUIN BOOKS

# DISCLAIMER

The information in this book is for educational purposes, and is written to inform readers about traditional remedies and methods in herbal medicine from around the world and to teach them to grow some of these plants in their gardens. It is not a replacement for professional medical advice. Many herbs are considered unsafe for pregnant women. Where possible, I have indicated these in the text, but whether you're using a remedy from this book or from any other sources, contact your midwife, doctor or a herbalist first if you are trying to conceive, or are pregnant or breastfeeding.

Likewise, if you are on any medication, prescribed or not, seek advice before you supplement or add home remedies. Finally do not use any remedies on children under two without checking with a herbalist or healthcare practitioner first.

nies

First published 2019

001

Copyright © Alys Fowler, 2019

The moral right of the author has been asserted

Set in 13.5/17pt Garamond MT Std
Typeset by Jouve (UK), Milton Keynes
Printed in Italy by Printer Trento Ltd S.r.l.

A CIP catalogue record for this book is available from the British Library

HARDBACK ISBN: 978–0–241–36833–6

www.greenpenguin.co.uk

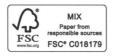

MIX
Paper from
responsible sources
FSC® C018179

Penguin Random House is committed to a sustainable future for our business, our readers and our planet. This book is made from Forest Stewardship Council® certified paper.

# INTRODUCTION

My journey with herbs started when I was very young, when my father, a physician, thought it was a worthwhile activity to teach all his children how to score opium poppies to collect morphine! Thankfully my mother, who is the grower in our family, taught me many more child-friendly ways with herbs: which plants to eat, which to rub on a sting, which to stroke for their lovely scent. I've always been a curious grower, ready to nibble, mash or crush a plant to find out more about it, but it wasn't till I went to New York that herbs became an integral part of my life.

When I was training as a horticulturist I got the opportunity to work and study at the New York Botanical Garden. Back then NYBG had a small herb garden to the left of the main greenhouse and the woman who looked after it was a self-proclaimed witch. She loved those herbs. US healthcare is notoriously expensive, so it was widely known that if you had a medical complaint, you went to the herb garden to ask her for a remedy before you went to the doctor. She gave me plants to chew on for a toothache and cramp-bark tea for period pains. When I got really sick, knowing I couldn't afford the upfront payments on my health insurance, someone in the East Village tipped me off about a Chinese herbalist who worked in a pharmacy. He prescribed cheap herbs and doled out warm and wonderful advice on how to use them. He rid me of heavy chest infections and persistent coughs with strange-tasting, bitter teas that cost me a fraction of antibiotics. When I look back on it now I came to herbs in a time-old tradition, seeking wisdom from those that grew and processed plants.

Herbs are useful plants, not just for us but for the ecosystem. They are good for insects, particularly the pollinators and beneficial creatures that are needed to keep your garden healthy. Herbs tend to have long flowering periods with nectar- and pollen-rich flowers. Think of how many bees you see visiting lavender, borage or rosemary, how many moths and hoverflies love marjoram and lemon balm. Many herbs have been bred by nature rather than artificially cultivated by humans and are therefore intrinsically linked to the ecology around them. A garden that feeds insects will be rich in other wildlife that comes to feed on those insects.

At the heart of all my gardening is a deep desire to create a place that supports the others in this world. I want my garden to feed me and all that visit it, whether they are blue tits or beetles. It is not so much of a leap then to arrive at my desire to grow herbs not just for the insects but for myself; for if these plants can keep my personal slice of the ecosystem healthy, then I am naturally curious as to how they might keep my internal ecosystem healthy too.

A year ago I was made president of the Herb Society and this brought me in touch with wonderful herb enthusiasts, medicinal herbalists, growers and practitioners. It's a place rich with shared knowledge and ideas. Through the Herb Society I was introduced to Hilda Leyel, our founder and author of numerous books on the subject of herbs. Leyel founded the society in 1927, with the aim of supporting herbal practice in Britain. She opened her own herbal shop, which was a huge hit, and campaigned tirelessly to keep herbal medicine relevant and widely available. In the 1940s the Pharmacy and Medicines bill threatened to make practising herbalism illegal, but Leyel successfully fought for its legitimacy. If you walk into a health food shop and buy any herbs to heal, whether that's echinacea or devil's claw, it's thanks in part to her. She also joined the pioneering agriculturist Sir Albert Howard in campaigning for organic growing methods after the Second World War and even set up a precursor to the National Lottery. A formidable woman indeed!

Thanks to women like Leyel, we have a vibrant herbal scene that continues today. Although there are many celebrated male herbalists, from the father of botany Theophrastus to ancient Greek physicians, such as Galen and Hippocrates, and John Gerard in the 1500s, there are many more women who kept the herbal tradition alive. These women have historically been hidden behind domesticity, their names lost, but through childcare, cooking and cleaning, home-birthing, breastfeeding, gardening, farming and foraging, ordinary women have passed down the magic of herbs for centuries. When my mother taught me where the lemony tang of sheep's sorrel leaves could be found in the meadows, she wasn't just directing me to a forageable snack, but keeping me healthy with a plant loaded with vitamins, trace minerals and tannins.

# A potted history of herbs

The dominant voice in herbalism is often rooted in Western traditions. Of course, Chinese and Ayurvedic practices are widely known and are referenced in this book, but in any history it's vital to ask who is telling the story. There's an equally long history of herbalism in black healing and indigenous peoples, Hispanic, Slavic, Mongolian and Tibetan cultures – indeed, around the world – for as long as there have been humans on a land they have used plants. Often when people cite one style of medicine they don't know that there's an equally long history somewhere else that uses the same herbs. Many herbal practices are largely oral traditions and because they have not been written down or referenced they may be ignored or discredited. There is a vast world of plant practices out there that many traditional histories of herbs neglect.

Growing herbs and practising your ancestral herbal traditions can be seen as a way to take back control of the dominant narrative of European or repackaged indigenous practices. It was only in researching this book that I learnt that ashwagandha, for example, has an equally long history in indigenous African herbalism as it does in Ayurvedic medicine. On both a personal and spiritual level your ancestral herbal practices might just work better for you, and this can be seen as claiming control over definitions of personal healthcare and resisting narratives that a certain herb or medicine is the 'best' method.

This of course presumes you know your ancestral heritage, which isn't always the case. This is perhaps the wonderful thing about herbal medicine, because although there are many branches to this tree, they all have the same roots in our most ancient of ancestors, the early humans who chewed on barks and roots and mashed leaves into poultices and cures. This certainly isn't about cultural appropriation of herbal traditions but respecting the long-held relationship between our species and the plant kingdom.

We sit here on this earth not only because we mastered language or evolved opposable thumbs but because plants provided a habitat for us to breathe in, made the soil for us to harvest our food, fed us, clothed us, sheltered us and healed us. Our first medicines were plants and fungi. Archaeological evidence that dates as far back as the Palaeolithic era has found plant quantities too small to be intended as food, seeds in the teeth of skeletons, symbolic depictions and fossilized sediments, all of which indicate the medicinal use of plants. The first known herbal remedies were found in southern Iraq, in what was ancient Sumer in southern Mesopotamia, and were written by the Sumerians, one of the earliest civilizations in the world. These 5,000-year-old recipes were written in cuneiform and carved into clay tablets. Of the roughly 30,000 tablets that the Sumerians left, over 1,000 of them deal with medical practices and include recipes for drug preparations for more than 250 different plants. These are sophisticated recipes showing an understanding of plant constituents such as the alkaloids in poppies and henbane. Around the sixth century BCE the first Ayurvedic scriptures appear. The earliest was written by a man known as Charaka, considered the Indian father of medicine. He was an early proponent of the 'prevention is better than cure' doctrine. He is attributed with writing, 'A physician who fails to enter the body of a patient with the lamp of knowledge and understanding can never treat diseases. He should first study all the factors, including environment, which influence a patient's disease, and then prescribe treatment. It is more important to prevent the occurrence of disease than to seek a cure.' A profoundly holistic approach. It is said that he was one of the first physicians to present the idea of digestion, metabolism and immunity.

Another important Ayurvedic text was written by Sushruta and is the oldest treatise dealing with surgery. Sushruta is known popularly as the father of surgery and the text indicates he was probably the first surgeon to perform plastic surgery, reconstructing a nose as well as carrying out cataract surgery. He mentions around 700 plants and how to use them to treat diseases, along with formulas for many plant medicines.

At roughly the same time ancient Egyptians made their own plant-based medicines. Around 1550 BCE the Papyrus Ebers was written, documenting around 700 plants, minerals and animal species that were used for medicine and over 800 recipes. It's thought that it may have been copied from older texts, but no one actually knows who wrote it and it remains one of the oldest and most significant papyri to have been found in ancient Egypt. It contains some inventive cures, like the treatment for guinea-worm disease, where you wrap the emerging end of the worm round a stick and slowly pull it out, which is still used today, as well as some less useful ones, such as using dates and honey for birth control and drinking beer-swill mixed with cucumber flowers and green dates for diabetes.

The earliest evidence of Chinese herbal medicine dates back to around 200 BCE. The first known Chinese herbal was written by a mythological deity, a venerated sage and ruler of prehistoric China called Shen Nung (or Shennong) in around 250 BCE. He is said to have experimented with hundreds of herbs to test their medicinal value, which he recorded in a book known as *The Divine Farmers' Herb-Root Classic*. It is said that he died of a toxic overdose from eating too much of a poisonous plant. His work is considered the basis of traditional Chinese herbalism and is probably a compilation of an even older oral tradition.

And then of course there were the Greeks, whose period in history has generally been considered the beginning of our Western medicine, though it is important to remember that Greek knowledge was garnered from the far corners of the world, from Alexander the Great's travels to Asia, India and Persia, as well as from local knowledge. Theophrastus created a system to classify more than 500 medicinal plants and wrote one of the first guides to gradual dosing, by which the dose of medicine is continually adjusted in response to the patient until the desired effect is achieved. This was a hugely important concept when so many of the plants used were poisonous (an idea that might have saved Shennong!).

The next notable contributor to the herbal tradition was Dioscorides who was born in what is now Turkey in around CE 40. He was a physician, pharmacologist and botanist, who travelled widely with the Roman military and wrote *De Materia Medica*, which offers plant descriptions, foraging information, guidance on how to express plants for their juice, concentrate them in the sun and store for future use. His book formed the basis for Western medicine for the next 1,500 years and was translated into multiple languages well into the sixteenth century, until it started to become supplanted by revised Renaissance herbals. In fact, Sir Arthur Hill, director of Kew Gardens, recorded that he saw a monk on Mount Athos using Dioscorides' texts to identify plants in 1934, making it one of the longest-lasting of all natural history books.

The post-classical era is commonly known in Europe as the Dark Ages, yet things were golden in the Arab world. Islamic medicine was advancing fast, integrating practices from ancient Greek, Roman, Persian and Ayurvedic traditions. This was all happening as much of western Europe lost its knowledge of classical medicine. During this period Europe was deeply unsettled, Barbarian tribes roamed over western Europe and many books of the Greek and Roman traditions were lost, burned or destroyed and the knowledge they contained replaced by speculation and superstition; students of medicine were judged not on scientific proof but debating skill, and to give you some flavour of that, a thirteenth-century Italian doctor called Alderotti claimed that combing the hair 'comforts the brain'.

European physicians only regained this classical knowledge when they became familiar with Islamic medical authors during the Renaissance. The original classical texts had been written in Greek, which for centuries had been the language of scholarship in the Mediterranean region, though many of these were also translated into Syriac, Arabic and Persian. During the Middle Ages many of these original texts were lost, but the translations weren't, and as the Arabic caliphate began to absorb Greek and Roman knowledge there was a shift in intellectual learning from Greek to the medieval Islamic world, particularly Arabic scholarship. Latin translations of Arabic works began what we now know as the Renaissance. It's odd to think that the knowledge to translate Greek was lost in the Middle Ages, but the Greek language almost died off along with the Roman Empire in the West, and by CE 500 very few people in western Europe were able to read or translate Greek text. Arabic scholars translated the famous authors of classical antiquity, including Hippocrates, Galen and Dioscorides. The Arabic world also made huge advances in surgery, and established and developed hospitals, and had female doctors, physicians, surgeons and midwives.

There are no more significant mentions of women in medicine until the eleventh century and the polymath Hildegard of Bingen. Among her achievements Hildegard wrote beautiful music, poetry and philosophy, and she is also considered the founder of scientific natural history in Germany. She was an abbess in a Benedictine monastery where she had a typical monastic herbal garden and helped to heal the sick. She wrote two major works on her healing practices, including the nine-book *Physica* that documented the various medical properties of plants, animals and stones, and *Causae et Curae*, which examined human healing through its connections to the rest of natural world. Hildegard believed that there was a vital connection between the green health of the natural world and the holistic health of a person. She approached her medicine as a type of gardening, with plants and elements of the garden grown as direct counterparts to elements of the human body. These books are historically hugely significant because they document medieval medicine in a time when its practitioners, who were mostly women, rarely wrote in Latin, if they could write at all.

During the fifteenth to eighteenth centuries herbalism boomed in all sorts of extraordinary ways. Before this time the printing press manuscripts were hand-copied, introducing many human errors along the way, but with the printing press came numerous self-proclaimed authoritative guides on using plants for medicine, from names such as John Gerard, Nicholas Culpeper and botanist Carl Linnaeus. By the early nineteenth century there was a huge shift in the medical industry, from plant-based medicines to organic chemicals. Instead of folk remedies and the traditional use of medicinal plants, chemists started to exploit the organic elements present in plants and create compounded medicines. Or, to put it another way, the shift moved away from making a tincture or tea of meadowsweet containing salicylic acid to creating a synthetic version in the form of the aspirin pill.

During the 1900s medical associations and new parliamentary bills, such as the one that Hilda Leyel fought against in 1941, proclaimed what was and wasn't medicine, how it should be labelled, distributed and used. All of these things were important for the burgeoning areas of manufacturing, administrating and teaching, but often herbs were routinely dismissed in favour of chemical drugs. The advent of antibiotics in the 1930s ushered in a new era and medicine firmly moved from botany to chemistry. These new chemical medicines changed lives forever and vastly increased lifespans. Herbalism began to fall by the wayside, mostly practised by those who didn't have access to or the means to pay for modern hospitals or doctors. By the 1950s the practice of teaching plants as medicine was almost dying out.

Herbalism saw a resurgence in the 1960s with the back-to-the-earth movement and this revitalization can be credited with our interest today. Modern herbalism now walks the tightrope between a clinically verifiable, evidence-based approach and the acknowledgement of a spiritual side, which suggests that plants have meaning beyond classification or their chemical constitutes, that they possess something significant to us that is both due to and other than their physical properties. You could see this as symbolic; think of the many ways we use plants ritually, even today, in the simple act of giving flowers or laying them on a grave. Or, in the greater meaning of biophilia, the hypothesis that humans possess an innate tendency to seek connections with nature, that our love of life helps to sustain life. We love plants because we need them.

As a feminist I have learnt a great deal from dipping into centuries' worth of herbal books. What struck me over and over again is that herbalism is a people's medicine. But it is also a medicine deeply nuanced in women's history. Never have I learnt so much about how to encourage breast milk to flow or how to wean a baby, of the subtle difference of period pains, the nuances of menopause or how to soothe weary, anxious, fretful children.

One way of understanding herbalism's popularity is to see it as a more intuitive method of everyday healthcare rather than a set of miracle cures. It seems that bodily autonomy and the skill to heal yourself is still a radical act. Herbalism is an appealing alternative to the one-solution-fits-all, disease-driven, dogma-laden and often paternal aspects of modern medicine. When you grow herbs to aid digestion, soothe a headache or boost your immune system, you are focusing on how to change your own life and health, on bodily autonomy. And no small part of that autonomy is that you grew them – all that advertising, plastic packaging, transportation costs, workers' rights, the whole shebang of capitalism, is nicely shook up by you nibbling on feverfew or brewing up some Californian poppy tea. That you can pass this knowledge freely to those around you is a radical idea in a world where much of the everyday medicine we use is dominated by ownership and branding. Just take a look at the wildly varying prices for paracetamol, which depend on whether it's a brand name or not; legally they are all required to have exactly the same amounts of active chemicals. Herbal manufacturing might be corporate, but the mint in your garden remains unbranded and free to anyone who can take a cutting to root in water.

For my part I come to growing herbs as I do to growing food. These are things my body needs, not just for hunger or to cure or alleviate, but to tend, pick and process. I get as much out of growing herbs as I do eating or using them. From sowing the seed to plucking the flower, I've been with these plants all the way. I've seen them struggle or thrive, coaxed them and adapted their ways. Working with herbs is hugely rewarding. I hope in some small way this book will encourage you to try growing something you might have previously bought from a health shop, to experiment with herbs in your cooking and bathing, or to see your weeds in a new light.

# ABOUT THIS BOOK

Before we proceed, let me lay out my wares. I want this guide to increase your confidence to experiment with your herbs, to reach into your garden before you pop open a blister pack. I want to show you how easy everyday herbalism is, how it is mostly an extension of eating, because food is our first medicine, and that many of the herbs you already use, whether that's as camomile or mint tea or chilli to spice your food, you can grow yourself.

I love eating, taking a bath and drinking tea. I truly love an afternoon nap. I am not so good at remembering to take tablets or tinctures or, for that matter, standing up straight. In short, I like doing things that are pleasurable and have a weak resolve for those things that are less so. This idiosyncratic guide is about the herbs that I love and therefore grow in my garden, and a few that I forage, and how I use them.

I like very simple recipes that I can make easily and quickly, which is why this herbal guide doesn't have a single tincture in it. This could be considered either a glaring error or a profound insight. Personally I take a tincture for a week and then forget the routine. Herbal tinctures use alcohol to extract the chief constituents of a plant, which is a charged and efficient way to concentrate the best of the plant into a few drops. There are many brilliant books and practitioners that can help you on that journey, but when using herbs I prefer to drink teas or add plants to a bath. It's the easiest and most enjoyable way to boost your well-being.

This book is not a medicinal guide and I have included a list of books for further reading in the Bibliography (see page 291). Everyone reacts differently to herbs, and medicinal herbalists tailor treatments to the client. It is possible to teach yourself a great deal about herbs and their medicine, but ultimately you need to be trained by professional herbalists who have extensive knowledge, experience and practice before you can treat yourself or others. I am not a trained herbalist; I am a gardener who uses herbs. The herbs in this book are ones I have used myself, so if you wonder why a certain herb is missing, it's because I don't have a comprehensive knowledge about growing or using it for myself.

Like I've said, I want you to think of your garden before your medicine cabinet for basic ailments and everyday woes. Instead of relying on over-the-counter sleeping pills, chemical pain relief, indigestion tablets, plastic plasters or petroleum-based creams, I want you to feel confident enough to reach for a few leaves or flowers from your garden first. For years I relied on painkillers for a hangover; now I reach first for liquorice mint for tea, which soothes my stomach and dulls my thumping head far more effectively (see page 134 – and refer to the chart at the end of the index for a full list of common ailments). Medicinal herbs can help many people with long-term complaints, such as depression, or recovery from serious illnesses, but you need to see a registered professional. In short, be sensible about how you use herbs; be mindful of their powers and careful with their ways.

# PREPARATION OF HERBS

Herbs are wonderful things, bringing in pollinators and beneficial insects, adding their notes of beauty to your garden, swaying in the wind and all that, but if you are to make the most of them, then you will have to pick and process them. Even if that's as simple as plucking a plantain leaf, chewing it up and spitting it out on to an insect bite or nettle sting. The wonder of herbs does not happen merely by looking at them.

Each herb has its moment when it needs to be picked. A camomile plant is not much use until it is in flower, and even then there is an art to when to pick the flowers so that they are open but don't immediately shatter on drying. There are nuances to all of these herbs and the truth is that experience is far more important than rules. You will learn when you process herbs that all plants are individuals responding to their environment and your growing techniques differently, and therefore you have to cut and pluck and pick with all your senses awake and alert. Look for moulds under leaves, look for damage and insects, note how the sun or shade affects the smell, feel, texture, thickness and taste of the plant. With careful observation you will quickly learn how and when you need to pick from your garden and how quickly you have to respond to changing weather.

This is part of the tradition of using herbs, to have a knowledge that is specific to your place in the world and using that over any rule about this or that.

# Drying herbs

Most fresh herbs contain around about 60–85 per cent water. Roots and rhizomes have a larger proportion of dry matter than leaves and flowers. By the time a herb has been successfully dried it should contain somewhere between 8–10 per cent water, though this can vary. You want the leaves to be dry enough that they don't turn mouldy, but not so dry that they are brittle and break when handled. This may mean experimenting around your house to find a place that is dry, warm and airy to dry the herbs quickly enough that you can achieve this. Kitchens, airing cupboards, above the fridge (which is always warm from the cooling system behind it) or near it are ideal. On top of the radiator doesn't work because of the swing of temperature.

One solution is to make or buy a herb-drying rack that can be suspended somewhere warm and airy. These are often made of material such as mesh frames and offer several shelves on which to dry. When not in use they are easily stacked for storage. If the summer is being kind and the weather is hot, then drying outside is often the perfect solution. You may need to cover your set-up with mesh netting to keep insects away, and all herbs should always be dried away from direct sunlight as the volatile oils in them are often easily destroyed by direct heat. If you find that you are processing a lot of herbs, then a dehydrator is invaluable. This will dry your herbs at a regulated temperature of 35°C/95°F. You can dry herbs at up to 46°C/115°F, and roots can be dried at up to 65°C/150°F.

If you are tying herbs in bundles to suspend from a hanger, make sure the bundles have sufficient space between them so that air can circulate. One solution is to create an indoor clothes line for your herbs and, using pegs, attach them individually to dry.

Your herbs are ready for storage when they feel paper-dry and they rustle. Under gentle pressure they will break up, but they're not brittle at a mere touch. Stems should not bend; if you squeeze the material gently and it reforms, there is still too much moisture.

Once dry your herbs need to be stored in an airtight container and kept out of direct sun. Some herbs, such as hops, will need to be kept in the fridge to maintain their properties, and no herb should be kept for such a long time that you can't remember when you picked it. As with all preserving techniques, date the container. If you do this, you can also start to monitor how much of a certain herb you need. If you've still got most of last year's supply, then you need to either grow or process less. If you've run out by December of a September harvest, you need to up your growing game. Of course, you can also go and buy dried herbs – there are plenty of reputable growers and suppliers.

If you have found that you didn't dry your herb sufficiently and they smell slightly mouldy, or you can see mould, then bin them rather than trying to re-dry them. The moulds that form on plant material are not necessarily harmful, but they are not something you need to drink or ingest.

# Infusions and decoctions

## How to make a cup of herbal tea

I never thought I'd write this, but there turns out to be a right and a very wrong way to make herbal tea. Our grandmothers made tea properly in a pot; we, the children of convenience and mass-produced teabags, make tea terribly, and it's nothing to do with how strong it looks. It's about capturing the volatile oils that do all the magical stuff.

There are two types of tea for herbs, an infusion or a decoction. Decoction refers to gently simmering your herbs in boiling water, and tends to be used with material that is tougher, such as roots, barks and seeds. An infusion is simply a cup of tea made by steeping the leaves, flowers and non-woody parts of the plant in either hot or cold water.

You can use fresh or dried herbs. Tear or cut up whole leaves to open the cell structures and release the chemical constituents. You will, however, have to use a greater volume of fresh herbs than dried to compensate for the higher water content. If you find instructions calling for one part dried herbs, say 1 teaspoon, then you will need to use three parts fresh herbs, as in 3 teaspoons. Or, put another way, 1 teaspoon of dried herbs equals 1 tablespoon of fresh. The truth of the matter is that a teaspoon can vary vastly depending on whether you crush, grind or chop the herb, but in weight terms you are looking for 1g of dried herbs or 3g of fresh herbs in a cup of water, which for ease I have made 250ml, because, let's face it, everyone's cups are slightly different.

Warm your teapot or cup by swilling some boiling water around in it, then disperse this. To save water I put this in my watering can for my houseplants, knowing by the time I get round to watering it will be cool. If you are making a pot, use 1 teaspoon of dried herb for each cup. Add 1 cup of water, 250ml, for each teaspoon of herbs in the pot and put the lid on immediately. If you are making a single cup, place a saucer on top. This bit is the most important part of the whole process; all those volatile oils are being lost to the air around if you don't do this. The more aromatic the herb is, the more volatile oils there are to lose.

The tea should be steeped for 10–15 minutes. You can drink the tea hot or cold, sweetened with honey or not. For medicinal purposes hot tea is usually recommended.

If you are using seeds and don't wish to make a decoction, then bash the seeds a little before making the tea, as this will release the volatile oils from the cells.

## Cold infusions

Another alternative is to make a cold infusion or a sun tea, where the herbs used are in the same concentration as hot tea but are left for 6–12 hours in a sealed pot or jar. I use large Kilner jars for this. I often leave the tea on a warm windowsill so that the sun can naturally brew the infusion. This tea never tastes as strong as tea made with boiling water, but it is refreshing and just as healthful. Cleavers with some added lemon or cucumber is particularly refreshing. I also like a nettle infusion made the same way (see page 199) and often find making litre batches an easier way to consume the herb than hot tea. Likewise, marshmallow is much better made in a cold infusion than hot as more of the active constituents are present this way (see page 170).

## Decoctions

Decoctions are for tougher, woody or hard material that just won't get broken down by hot water alone. Roots, rhizomes, wood, bark, nuts and some seeds have such strong cellular walls that they need a little vigorous action to ensure that the active constituents actually end up in the water. A simple method is to put 1 teaspoon of dried herbs (or 3 teaspoons of fresh material) in a saucepan, add the appropriate amount of water, which will be a little more than for a cup of tea as some will be lost to evaporation. Bring to the boil and simmer for 10–15 minutes, if possible with a lid on the pot, so that you don't lose any volatile oils. Strain the tea while hot. If you are making a mixture with both tough and softer herbs, simmer the tough herbs separately and combine if possible, because boiling leaves and flowers for 15 minutes will mean you've very little left of the softer parts.

## Baths

There is only so much tea a person can drink, and when that point comes consider having a bath because many of the herbal teas can be absorbed in a nice long soak, and it can have just as good an effect as drinking the tea. You can make your bath using either a concentration of tea or decoction anywhere between 500ml and a litre (2–4 cups) or you can take a handful of herbs and place them in a muslin bag that you suspend under the hot-water tap. If you don't have any muslin, just tie a cotton hanky round the flower heads or seeds. If you decide to do away with the bag and scatter your petals for a more romantic look, have a strainer in the plughole or you'll end up with a blocked drain (not so romantic).

You can add Epsom salts to your herbal bath. Epsom salts help to draw out impurities in the skin and increase circulation. They can help with bedsores, aches and pains and can also relieve itching. Likewise, sea salt can also be added to improve skin tone and as a natural antiseptic.

Fragrant, relaxing bath herbs include lavender, camomile, calendula, lemon balm, rosemary and lime flowers. For a bath that is truly sedative try adding Valerian roots and rhizomes, but note it does have a very strong smell.

For teething babies and children who won't sleep, camomile and lime flowers are both suitable.

For colds, flu and when you need to sweat something out, try yarrow, chilli, rosemary or ginger. For very obvious reasons you should only use tiny amounts of chilli and ginger, and some might prefer to try these as a footbath or hand bath. Surprisingly both foot and hand baths work just as effectively as a whole bath, stimulating the whole system.

---

### Herbs for decoctions

| | | |
|---|---|---|
| Angelica root | Caraway seed | Echinacea root |
| Barberry dried fruit | Dandelion root | Elecampane |
| Burdock root | Dill seed | Liquorice |

---

### Herbs for infusions

| | | |
|---|---|---|
| Angelica | Chickweed | Fennel |
| Blackberry | Chilli | Feverfew |
| Calendula | Cleavers | Goldenrod |
| Californian poppy | Dandelion | Heartsease |
| Camomile | Dill | Hops |
| Caraway | Elderberry | Juniper |
| Celery | Eucalyptus | Lady's mantle |

| | | |
|---|---|---|
| Lemon balm | Oats | Sage |
| Lime blossom | Parsley | St John's wort |
| Marshmallow | Plantain | Sweet violet |
| Meadowsweet | Raspberry | Thyme |
| Mint | Red clover | Valerian |
| Mullein | Rosemary | Wild lettuce |
| Nettle | Rue | Yarrow |

# Poultices and compresses

I love the idea that there are plants in my garden as good as a sticking plaster. As someone who regularly fails to remember to wear gardening gloves, my hands show the scars of years of work. I'm very happy to reach for a soft leaf of pelargonium and to mash up some selfheal or plantain to draw out that painful splinter. Plus, at the end of the whole thing, my mashed-up plant poultice can go on the compost or be flushed down the loo (and we all know how revolting old plasters are).

Now it is worth saying that the conventional plaster is a thing of genius and by no means am I suggesting that if you hack into yourself you should go and wrap up your gaping wound with a leaf. Be practical. It's just if you have a stubborn thorn, an insect bite or sting, a minor scrape or a whitlow that won't heal, trying a little mash-up of plants, even if it is under a plaster, is worth a go. Be sensible: prepare the plant material in a manner so that it's clean and not going to introduce anything unpleasant. When making a poultice make sure to clean the wound under running water before using the herbs, just the way you would before applying a regular plaster. When the leaves go black it's time to replace them with a clean batch. This might be far more often than you'd replace a shop-bought plaster. Be wise, and don't pursue a remedy that's not working. If your cut/wound/scrape isn't healing from the plant mash, stop using it.

## Poultices

To prepare a poultice, mash or crush fresh plant material mixed with a little hot water to make a paste. If you are using dried herbs, powder them in a pestle and mortar or grinder before mixing with water to make a paste. Apply directly to the skin, either hot or cold. You can hold the poultice in place with gauze or clean cotton or muslin strips. I often use micropore tape. If you are using stimulating herbs, such as mustard, apply between two layers of cloth.

## Compresses

A compress differs from a poultice in that it uses liquid, rather than fresh or dried plant material. A poultice is a stronger form of applying herbs to a minor infection, wound or swelling, but compresses can be very good for relieving muscle tension. To make a compress soak a clean linen or cotton cloth in hot herbal tea and apply it to the affected part of the body. I often use compresses to relieve headaches and sinus pain or round the back of my neck to alleviate stress. Use the compress as hot as can be tolerated and cover with a clean, dry towel to hold in the heat. When cool replace with a fresh compress for another round. You can also make a cool compress, which is sometimes favourable for headaches; use exactly the same method but allow the infusion to cool before applying.

# Herbs to heal cuts, minor wounds, grazes

Chickweed is very healing to any wound, including minor burns, and is soothing enough for skin irritations (see page 72).

Comfrey root – dried and powdered and turned into a paste – should not be used on puncture wounds or deep, infected injuries, but it is good for repairing strains and torn muscles and tendons (see page 57). Or you can use the fresh whole plant: you chop the clean scrubbed root with an equal part of green comfrey leaves, blending them to a paste with a little water, and spreading them over the injured area and covering with a clean cloth. It is best applied at night and then cleaned off the following day. Comfrey is known as knit-bone for its healing properties for internal strains and bruises.

Geranium leaves, the soft leaves of scented pelargoniums, are gentle enough to be used as a plaster to keep a cut supple and help healing.

Herb Robert – a poultice of washed roots and leaves can help relieve bruises and swelling. A fresh leaf will act as a styptic and stem bleeding. It's a good one if you cut yourself in the garden as the crushed leaf will stem minor bleeding very quickly.

Lady's mantle (see page 136) – the young leaves can be mashed into a poultice that is astringent and will stem bleeding. It is very good at preventing infection and was once widely used on the bat-tlefield along with yarrow (see below and page 283).

Plantain (see page 217) – mashed plantain leaves are very good at drawing out splinters, for infections and for soothing insect bites. If you keep bees, you'll find they are miraculous at stopping a bee sting from swelling.

Selfheal (see page 251) will draw out infections, and soothes and heals wounds. It's very good for insect bites and those stubborn scrapes that won't seem to heal.

Yarrow leaves (see page 283) are a wonderful astringent, stem bleeding and have good antiseptic properties. Either bruise or mash the leaves and use for quite deep cuts and scrapes as well as bruises. It is truly the go-to herb for first aid.

# Herb oils

As you might have guessed from a cursory glance at this work, I am into easy solutions. I am very happy eating my herbs and drinking them and even more so lying in a deep bath full of them. I am not afraid of mashing them up for poultices and compresses, but my patience wanes a little when it comes to complicated bottling or extraction processes. Which is why there aren't any tinctures in here, nor any recipes for creams and salves. It's not that I am lazy, just immediate about the business of my health. However, I do make an exception for herbal oils, made the folk way using the sun. These are so simple to make and there are a few that are genuinely invaluable medicines to have a ready supply of. These infused oils are not suitable for culinary purposes.

Herbal oils should not be confused with essential oils or hydrosols that are made by distilling the plant materials to capture the volatile oils of a herb. Nor are they medicinal herb oils that extract all the physical constituents of a plant into an oil base. Herbal oils are made by infusing herbs into an oil base, much like you might infuse herbs into a vinegar for cooking. The oil is most usually olive oil, but you can experiment with almond, avocado, jojoba, grapeseed, apricot, castor or coconut oil. As these herb-infused oils are all pre-pared at a low heat, any base oil can be used that suits your skin and needs best.

I have very sensitive skin and have learnt over time that what works best for me is to use as few ingredients as possible. Herbal oils work wonderfully for my skin because of this. They certainly don't have the sophistication of shop-bought stuff and aren't grease-free, but they are readily absorbed, kind to children's skin and, if you use a base like grapeseed oil, full of natural antioxidants.

Any jar used for herbal oil needs to be sterilized first. This is important as it ensures that there is no contamination in your oil. To do this first wash the jar thoroughly in hot soapy water, before rins-ing and draining. Then place the jar on an oven rack with space between jars, if making batches, and heat at 120°C/250°F for 10–15 minutes. Ensure the jar is completely dry before adding liquid. Alternatively you can put the jars in a large pot of boiling water for 10 minutes. Let the water cool and then remove. Let the jars drain upside down on a clean tea towel. If using Kilner jars, boil the rubber seals as dry heat damages them.

## The folk method

The simplest way to make a herbal oil is using what's known as the folk method. This uses a paper bag as the only heat source to raise the temperature a tiny bit.

Half fill a rubber-sealed preserving jar (a Mason jar is ideal) with dried, coarsely ground herbs. If you are using fresh herbs, fill them almost all the way to the top. Add your chosen oil to reach the top of the jar and with a clean utensil gently mix back in any material that floats to the top. Allow the contents to settle and gently tap or shake the jar to release any air bubbles that might be trapped. Place the jar in a paper bag and set in a warm place (18–25°C/64–77°F) – a sunny windowsill or a cupboard is perfect. Shake the container as often as you remember, ideally about twice a day, for 1–2 weeks. Strain the oil into another jar, secure the lid, and you can now let it sit for a further few days before straining through cheesecloth to remove any sediment. You can make a double strength oil by adding a second batch of herbs to your initial infusion for another 2 weeks. Once you've strained out any sediment, pour the herbal oil into a clean jar and store in a cool dry place. It should store for up to a year.

You can use dried or fresh herbs for this method, but there are a handful of herbs that must be processed fresh, which include Californian poppy (good for aiding restful sleep, see page 222), St John's wort (good for healing cuts and wounds, see page 261) and garlic (see page 108, but the method is not suitable for making garlic oil for consuming).

## The solar-infused method

This method is specifically for fresh herbs.

Before your herbs are infused in oil it is important that they wilt a little, so leave for 8–12 hours somewhere warm, but away from direct sunlight so that they do not completely dry.

Place the wilted herbs directly into the jar. You need roughly a one-to-five ratio of herbs to oil. Use a piece of cheesecloth to cover the mouth of the jar, but do not put the lid back on. Secure the cheesecloth with a rubber band. Leave the jar on a sunny windowsill for 2–3 weeks (the latter if the sun is not always out in your world) and shake the mixture daily. You may notice quite a lot of residue at the bottom of the jar. This is the water that is being extracted from the plants into the oil. It may be necessary to decant the oil into another vessel to remove this gunk, and you may have to do this several times. When the oil is ready strain through a cheesecloth and repeat this process until you have a residue-free oil. Decant this into a clean, dry jar and store it in a cool, dark place.

# ALOE

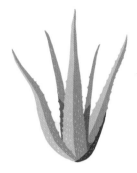

**Other Name** True aloe.

**Botanical Name** *Aloe vera.*

**Family** Asphodelaceae (lily family).

**Parts Used** Leaves.

**Plant Properties** Anti-inflammatory, antioxidant, antibacterial, immune-enhancing.

**Uses** All kinds of first- and second-degree burns, including sunburn, heat and chemical burns; dermatologically to cool and moisten dry skin; as a laxative.

**Preparations** Oral or topical gels.

**Considerations** The laxative effect of ingesting the sap means that it is not suitable for women who are pregnant or breastfeeding. It is a harsh laxative and should only be used after consulting a medical practitioner. If you have a known allergy to the lily family, Asphodelaceae, then you should also not use aloe either orally or topically as allergenic reactions may occur.

The true aloe, *Aloe vera,* originally comes from the Arabian peninsula, but it has been widely cultivated and, as a result of human distribution, has been naturalized across the world. Aloe was known to the Greeks as early as the fourth century BCE and is said to have been first cultivated on the island of Socotra in the Arabian Sea. Legends claim that Aristotle requested Alexander the Great to conquer the island in order to obtain the knowledge of how to grow and use the Socotrine aloes, which Aristotle believed to be a great purgative. It was widely naturalized along the banks of the Nile and it is said that Cleopatra used aloe as part of her beauty regime.

Aloe is a common cosmetic ingredient; you'll find it in everything from nail polish remover to facial tissues. Despite this, there's little conclusive medical research into its effectiveness. As someone who burns at the drop of sunlight and therefore spends a lot of time rubbing aloe in, I wonder in part if it's not studied because it's just so quietly useful.

There is a huge difference between aloe sap fresh from the plant and aloe gel. The shelf life of the mucilaginous sap contained in the flesh is very short and aloe gel contains preservatives in order to capture this. The very best results seem to occur when you use a fresh leaf directly on the skin.

## How to grow

*Aloe vera* is a popular houseplant that can be brought outdoors for the summer, but is not frost-tolerant, so will have to winter indoors. It is naturally found in the rocky, free-draining soils of deserts and the arid grassland of steppe landscapes. It needs good light and very free-draining but humus-rich soil to be happy. It's almost impossible to kill, unless you let it sit in water all day every day.

However, there's a big difference between a healthy aloe and one that's just holding on. A healthy aloe has plump, light green leaves with a slightly blueish hue; orange or pink tinges are signs of stress, with the former signalling sunburn. Despite being a succulent, aloe doesn't like full sun and its orange display is akin to putting on suntan lotion to protect its chlorophyll, the green parts of the cell that produce the energy. If your plant starts to turn yellow or orange, move it to part shade.

In order to grow plump, healthy leaves, it is important to feed your plant through the growing season – once a month is fine from May to October – and to repot the plant every three years or so. This way you'll get lots of 'pups', baby aloe plants that can be repotted to make new plants.

## How to use

### For topical use

The sap can be applied freely to the skin to moisten, cool and heal. Cut off a fat leaf and squeeze out the sap, much like you might a tube of toothpaste. If you find that you are not getting enough sap, then you can slice the leaf in half lengthwise and then, with a teaspoon, scrape out the gel right up to the rind where some of the best constituents can be found. It is said to be a very good cure for mastitis, but make sure to wash off any residue from the nipple to avoid laxative effects for the baby. For topical use apply up to three times a day until symptoms reduce.

Alternatively take a leaf, splice the outer tissues lengthways, then open the leaf up and use as a poultice, applying it to the affected area for around 20 minutes or so. This can be a particularly soothing medicine for burnt fingers. Poultices can be reused if wrapped in a plastic bag and left in the fridge, although they don't last much longer than a day.

## For oral use

Aloe sap can also be consumed orally. It can be a very strong laxative used to treat constipation. In my experience if your stomach is sensitive, it's too powerful and there are gentler alternatives. It is not suitable for long-term use. It is said that the laxative properties are found in the yellow latex to the edge of the leaf and the mid-pulp is mild. Use 250–450mg of the leaf sap, but a medical practitioner's advice is recommended.

# ANGELICAS

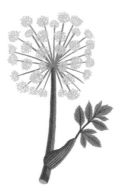

**Other Name**  Wild celery.

**Botanical Name**  *Angelica* species.

**Family**  Apiaceae (carrot family).

**Parts Used**  Roots (medicinal); leaves, stems and seeds (culinary).

**Plant Properties**  Astringent, tonic, diuretic, anti-inflammatory.

**Uses**  Expectorant for coughs; improves digestion; appetite-stimulant; antiseptic for urinary infections.

**Preparations**  *Angelica archangelica* is a common flavour for liqueurs and is used in gin, vermouth, chartreuse and Benedictine; candied stalks; tea made from seeds.

**Considerations**  Many plants in the Apiaceae family are photosensitive, meaning that if the sap gets on skin it can react to UV light, causing skin sensitivities. Wear gloves and long-sleeved shirts when harvesting this plant. High doses of angelica may interfere with anticoagulants. The root is nearly always used dried because fresh root may irritate mucous membranes.

**Angelica is not recommended for pregnant women.**

There's a good chance that you've been drinking plenty of angelica already; the roots and, in some cases, flowers and seeds have been traditionally used in gin for centuries. The flavour of the roots is earthy and bitter, somewhat reminiscent of wormwood, but with grassy herbal notes. The seeds taste a little more like juniper; there's something floral present, and, again, a grassy, almost nettle-like scent.

*Angelica archangelica* is not the only species in the genus that is much loved for these herbal properties. There are a number of species from Japan and Korea that have a long history of both culinary and medicinal uses. Ashitaba, *Angelica keiskei*, is native to the Pacific coast in Japan and is revered as a healthful ingredient that promotes long life. It is packed full of minerals and vitamins and has appreciable amounts of dietary fibre. It's nearly always grown from seed. The newly emerging leaf and stem are eaten, and the succulent leaf stem can be used much like celery or the young leaves used sparingly in salads. The leaves and stems can also be used in soups.

Asian angelica species have long been celebrated in their natural habitats as folk medicine. Dong quai, *Angelica sinensis*, is largely used in Korean and Chinese herbal medicine, where the root is used dried and often used in a tea to improve circulation, relax menstrual cramps and protect the liver. It is a laxative and not to be used during pregnancy. It grows well in dappled shade. Likewise, the beautiful *Angelica gigas*, dang-gui, is also used in Korean folk medicine for menstrual issues and overall gynaecological health. It's one of the most beautiful plants in my garden, offering architectural structure both in its leaves and its great dome of a flower head that is always crowned in hundreds of bees.

# How to grow

Angelicas are handsome plants from the carrot family that often tower to 1.8 metres or more, with impressive globe-shaped flowers and thousands of seeds. Most are biennial, meaning that they flower every second year and then, if allowed, liberally scatter seeds all over your garden. In a small garden this can result in an army of seedlings, but they are not difficult to weed out when young and once established rarely need to be manually re-sown; buy one plant, let it go to seed and you'll never have to replant. It is possible to grow angelicas in a pot, but, like carrots, they do need space for their long taproot (it is one of the characteristics of the carrot family to have a long, carrot-like root), so containers should be 5–10 litres in volume. Plants grown in pots may be much smaller than their in-ground counterparts because of root restriction. They grow best in well-drained, moist soil in sun, but can survive in partial shade. They are much loved by the pollinators and the flower heads teem with bees and hoverflies. Asian species, such as ashitaba and dang-gui, are more shade-tolerant.

# How to use

The aerial parts of *Angelica archangelica* are harvested prior to flowering and used fresh or dried. The roots should be harvested in the first year before the plant's autumn flowering. Seeds are harvested once they are mature and have turned buff-coloured.

## Angelica archangelica tea

The easiest way to use this herb is to make a tea from the seeds. You can drink this alone or add to other loose tea mixtures, where it will impart its gentle digestive properties. It is said to be good for colic, flatulence and constipation. Use 1 teaspoon of seeds with up to 1 cup of boiling water. As this tea is an aromatic bitter it's best to take before meals to improve digestion. The tea can warm and comfort colds and the flu, helping to boost immunity and soothe coughs.

You can also make a decoction of the root to drink as a tea. To do this, place 1 teaspoon of dried roots in 1 cup of water (250ml) and bring to the boil, allow to cool, and drink. This can be taken up to three times a day and, like the seeds, is very good for digestion. I will say this: it is not the most delicious-tasting drink. Given a choice, I go for the seeds for tea.

# ARTICHOKES

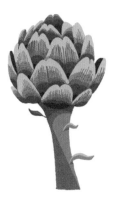

**Other Name** Cardoon.

**Botanical Names** *Cynara scolymus* (artichoke), *Cynara cardunculus* (cardoon).

**Family** Asteraceae (sunflower or daisy family).

**Parts Used** Flower heads, leaves.

**Plant Properties** Improves digestion, liver tonic.

**Uses** Culinary, teas, infusions.

**Preparations** Bitters, teas.

**Considerations** Some people are sensitive to the Asteraceae family and therefore should avoid artichokes. If you have a bile duct obstruction, then you should also avoid artichoke tea.

Oh! Majestic globe artichoke, the prince of the vegetable garden, handsome enough for the flower garden, architectural and stately in stature, to say nothing of the flavour of those flower buds. In truth, the artichoke is a pumped-up, supersized version of its ancestor, the wild thistle. It's an ancient vegetable with a long history of cultivation. The Romans and Greeks favoured it for both culinary and medicinal purposes. Its flavour is hard to pin down; the unopened flower head has the green tinge of asparagus, but also a hint of mushroom and perhaps the taste of the woodland floor.

You cannot mention artichokes without some nod to their wild cousin, the cardoon, *Cynara cardunculus*. The cardoon is a lankier version of the globe artichoke with taller flower stems and slightly smaller flower heads. It easily grows to 1.5 metres tall. Italians use cardoon stems in an oven-baked gratin, which is quite something, the nuttiness of the stem with a hint of bitter tempered by a good layer of parmesan cheese. Cardoon stems need to be blanched with a huge black bucket, bin or forcing pot, or else they are too bitter. They are peeled of their stringy midribs, much like overzealous celery stems, and soaked in salt water to further diminish the bitterness and, even then, the hint remains. I love bitter flavours, so all this effort for a few stems seems well worth it to me, but I will acknowledge that this bitterness, which becomes even more present in tea, is not going to be everyone's cuppa. Still, like many things in life, it is an acquired taste. Drink the tea over and over again and you will become fond of it, particularly as, when groaning after too much excess of other things, it soothes a sore belly.

The common globe artichoke is a delicious thing, but these days we tend to concentrate on eating the heart and give little thought to the rest of the plant, or for that matter to the leaves (sepals) that are discarded along the way. The heart is delicious, but the other parts are packed full of goodness, and since the Greeks, folk traditions have used artichokes to aid digestion and stimulate the production of bile in the liver, as well as the release of bile from the gallbladder. Bile is important in digestion as it breaks down fats, allowing us to absorb essential fat-soluble substances such as vitamins A, D, E and K. Whether you regularly suffer from bloating after eating or just ate a heavy meal, artichokes can help to stimulate your digestive system.

Artichokes are high in a phenolic acid, or cynarine, which can make everything, including water, taste sweet after it's consumed. It is disastrous for wine; it makes it taste like sweet vinegar, and not in a good way, which is why traditionally artichokes are served at the beginning of the meal, so you can wash away the cynarine with sweet water and move on to something a little stronger. It is thought that cynarine has beneficial properties for the liver. Another constituent is silymarin, which is also found in milk thistle and again is thought to be beneficial for the liver. Additionally many people believe artichoke tea does wonders for your skin due to its high anti-oxidant content. Several studies have also shown artichoke extracts to reduce cholesterol.

## How to grow

Artichoke is very easy to grow from seed and there are numerous varieties available, whereas young plants tend to be limited to the commercial American variety 'Green globe'. From seed the plants can be harvested in their second year, though in my experience it's the third year that they get into their stride. The seed is quickest started off on a warm windowsill in early spring and then hardened off in late spring when all chance of frost has passed. You will see quite a wide variation in seedling vigour and leaf colour. I select the most silvered leaves because I like that look in my garden. 'Violette' has violet-coloured petals in the flower head. 'Vert de Laon' is a particularly hardy variety, and 'Purple Sicilian' has very small purple heads that can be eaten raw when young.

Cardoon are very easy to grow, requiring less sun and even managing in poor, dry conditions. But if you want fat midribs for eating, then you'll need to give them more lush and fertile feet to get good growth. They require a long growing season of about five months, but as they are perennial this is little of an issue. The top growth is frost-sensitive, so situate them somewhere sheltered from the first frosts. If you want to grow perennially, rather than sowing seed each year, you will need to cut out the flowering stalk when it appears. You can then blanch the plants using a large black bin; the stalks are going to be at least 45cm long, so a bucket will not suffice nor wrapping them in newspaper packed with straw for several weeks. You need to prevent moisture building in the base of the plant or else the stems will rot or fill with slugs, hence why the black bin can be useful – it'll keep the rain off and stop the whole thing from rotting. You can also easily lift the bin off to check for marauding slugs.

If you have established perennial plants, you can bypass this faff and eat the young stems in spring, when the bitterness is barely present.

## How to use

There are two types of artichoke tea, one using the true leaves of artichoke and a folk-sourced recipe using the outer leaves (sepals) of the artichoke head. If you don't grow your own artichokes, then you'll have to order the true leaves from a herbalist. The folk recipe can be used with any artichoke heads, be it from the back garden or a shop.

## True leaf bitter artichoke tea

The true artichoke leaves pack an even more powerful punch than the outer sepals of the flower head. We've shied away from bitter tastes over the years, but the mouth-puckering flavour often accompanies foods that aid digestion. You can find artichoke tea already prepared from most health food shops, but if you grow artichokes, you'll have plenty of leaves to play with. This tea is a very good aid to digestion when drunk regularly.

Either cardoon or artichoke leaves can be used for this tea. I use the younger leaves towards the centre of the plant, which are generally in good health and free from any blemishes, mould or other types of damage. It is incredibly important not to dry any leaves that have any sort of mould growing on them (powdery or downy mildews). Harvest leaves before the flower bud appears in spring, taking a few leaves from each plant; this way you shouldn't exhaust the plant too much by taking its source of energy, so it should still flower. You may find more leaves to pick in autumn.

The leaves should be dried somewhere warm away from direct sun: a kitchen is ideal. I use a dehydrator, but it is possible to rig up a drying rack or just hang the leaves upside down high above a radiator. When drying any sort of leaf, use a low, steady heat source rather than blasting the leaves to avoid loss of potency and colour. Once the leaves are dry enough to crumble, store in a cool, dry place in a rubber-sealed preserving jar. Although the leaves don't go off, they will lose vitality with age, so use them up before the following spring.

## Artichoke leaf tea

This tea is best made in a teapot where the leaves can expand. Use a scant teaspoon of dried leaves per cup for tea, add boiling water and steep for at least 10 minutes. Then strain and add honey or sugar to taste. If using a cup or mug, cover with a saucer so that you don't lose too much goodness to evaporation. You can add fresh ginger, lemon verbena, lemongrass or lemon balm to temper the bitterness.

You can also make this tea with fresh leaves. As with all herbs, dried leaves are concentrated in goodness and can be stored (there are not going to be any fresh leaves to pick in the middle of winter). However, fresh leaves often have a different flavour and I think it's good to try out both fresh and dry to find the best fit for you. You'll also begin to notice how herbs taste at different times of the year; in spring there's a noticeable vitality that's not present by autumn, but instead the leaves might be sweeter or nuttier. I can't press upon you enough the joy in truly getting to know your plants day in, day out. There's a world of shifting and subtle flavours that the shops will never give you.

## Vietnamese iced tea

Numerous digestive tea recipes include artichoke, such as this Vietnamese iced tea, which often adds basil seed, pandan and dried loganberries with lump sugar. The simplest way to make the tea is to take a large artichoke head, slice it in half, cover with water and then boil for 30 minutes. Allow the water to cool and remove the head and enjoy, with or without honey or sugar, adding ice to serve. If you want to save the heart, you could just boil the artichoke as you would in preparation for eating it and save the cooking liquid to drink. Iced artichoke tea is delicious and works perfectly as an after-dinner bitter or between the main course and pudding. Alternatively drink before a meal to stimulate digestion. The cooking liquid can be stored in a rubber-sealed preserving jar in the fridge for several days.

## *Amaro di carciofi* digestif

The Italian aperitif Cynar is similar to Aperol (and often used in a Spritz), only more bitter. This is a home-made version. In small amounts (around 10–15 drops) it can be used as a bitter or digestif. In large amounts it's one hell of a powerful cocktail ingredient . . . You decide.

30 fresh, tender artichoke sepals from inside the flower head

3–5 artichoke stems, peeled (use the top half of the stem, nearest the flower head)

1 lemon

1 pinch cloves

1 litre vodka or gin.

The traditional recipe uses dry white wine and a brandy (five-to-one ratio). I prefer vodka, mostly because its clean flavour is an easy base to build on.

1 litre water

700g sugar

Wash and dry the sepals and peeled stems, which should be cut into 1cm pieces. Peel the lemon, making sure that you don't have any pith or white rind as this will make the already bitter infusion even more so. A potato peeler works excellently for this. Place the artichokes, stems, lemon rind and cloves in a large jar with a lid and cover with alcohol. Leave for 10–20 days. Shake the jar every so often to disperse the flavours. The liquid will have gone a brown colour. I suggest tasting after 10 days and seeing if the flavour is complex enough (remember until you add the sugar it's going to be very bitter).

When your alcohol is ready, make a sugar syrup with the water and sugar. Bring 1 litre of water to the boil and add the sugar, stirring constantly until it dissolves. When the syrup begins to boil, lower the heat and simmer for 10 minutes. Remove and let cool.

Add the sugar syrup to the alcohol, then strain with a muslin before sieving and bottling. Store the liqueur somewhere cool and dark and consume within 2–3 months.

# ASHWAGANDHA

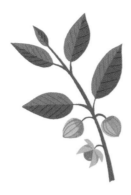

**Other Names** Indian ginseng, poison gooseberry, winter cherry.

**Botanical Name** *Withania somnifera.*

**Family** Solanaceae (nightshade family).

**Parts Used** Roots, aerial parts.

**Plant Properties** Energy-building, aphrodisiac, sedative, anti-inflammatory, antioxidant.

**Uses** Fresh aerial parts for poultices; roots for tea or decoctions; ground root as food supplement.

**Preparations** Poultices, powders, teas.

**Considerations** If you are sensitive to the Solanaceae family (which includes tomatoes and potatoes), bear in mind that ashwagandha may bring out your sensitivities. In Ayurvedic medicine ashwagandha is not used if there are upper respiratory infections or mucus; a qualified practitioner can advise best on this. The aerial part should never be eaten or used internally. The root is always used dried to reduce any potential side effects.

---

**Do not take ashwagandha during pregnancy unless you have consulted a qualified herbalist or doctor. Ashwagandha may have sedative effects, so avoid taking alongside barbiturates.**

---

Ashwagandha is a venerated herb that has been used for centuries in both Indian and African medicine. It has recently become a popular ingredient in Western herbalism, in part because of its infamy as a male aphrodisiac. Yet this herb does much more than that. Ashwagandha is used to strengthen the tired and weary, and calm the anxious and stressed, of whom there are more than ever.

Happily it's as easy to grow as a tomato. It needs a little heat in its early life and can successfully be grown in a pot, making it the perfect plant for a patio, warm courtyard or greenhouse, as well as suiting a sunny spot as a houseplant. It likes warmth and humidity so if grown outside in the ground, it needs to be a sheltered spot in full sun. It won't win prizes for its looks, though the ripening of the red cherries in their paper lanterns can attract some admiring glances.

The roots are the real champion of this plant. Once dried and powdered they can be added to food, such as smoothies, milk drinks or cereals. Studies have shown that taking the herb regularly promotes restful sleep, helps with day-to-day fatigue and lowers feelings of anxiety. It is high in antioxidants and it's thought that these are responsible for its effectiveness supporting sexual desire and fertility, particularly in men, where it is supposed to improve semen quality. A limited pilot study also showed that ashwagandha can boost female sexual health and improved orgasm.

Now, ashwagandha root is famed for smelling rather bad, like horse urine. For this reason it's mainly consumed in drinks or sweeter foods that can hide its bitter aromas and flavours. Warm, sweetened nut milks, golden milks, porridges, matcha lattes, raw cacao drinks and nut or date balls are just some of the many inventive recipes people have come up with to get their daily dose. In traditional Ayurvedic practices the ashwagandha is often mixed with ghee, honey and either trikatu powder (a blend of black pepper, long pep-per and ginger) or black pepper powder to increase the absorption of the herb.

## How to use

In the autumn, before the first frosts appear, dig up your plants, cut off the roots, wash them carefully, then leave them somewhere warm out of direct sunlight to dry. Once dried, blend the roots in a coffee grinder or food processor. The recommended dose is 3–6g a day, which is roughly ½ teaspoon.

# BASILS

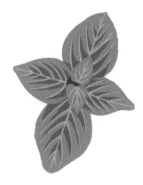

**Botanical Name** *Ocimum* species.
**Family** Lamiaceae (mint family).
**Parts Used** Leaves, seeds.
**Plant Properties** Antimicrobial, antiviral, antispasmodic, circulatory stimulant.
**Uses** Antibacterial, appetite-stimulant, improves digestion, stomach-soothing, relieves flatulence.
**Preparations** Baths, infusions, steam inhalations, teas.

**Considerations** None known for common basil. Holy basil may affect fertility in both men and women and regular consumption might not be ideal if you are trying to conceive. It has a slight ability to thin the blood and therefore anyone taking blood-thinning medicine, such as warfarin, should consult their doctor. It also lowers blood sugar and may affect people with diabetes.

A soft, sweet basil leaf wrapped round a sun-warmed, home-grown tomato must be one of the greatest pleasures in life. Or maybe torn across some burrata with a generous slug of good olive oil, garnishing a really good thin pizza or floating fragrant in a Thai soup. Basil's flavour is only truly captured when freshly picked and, as it grows year-round on a windowsill, it is the one herb you should always have to hand.

Basils are found in the mint family, Lamiaceae, and come originally from tropical and warm places. The two most well-known species are sweet basil, *Ocimum basilicum*, beloved by both the Greeks and Romans, and the sacred and medicinal holy basil or tulsi, *O. tenuiflorum*. There are numerous culinary cultivars and crosses: a basil that tastes of lemon, *O. × citriodorum*, or cinnamon, *O. basilicum* 'Cinnamon', or liquorice, *O. basilicum* 'Horapha', or the highly aromatic African blue basil, *O. basilicum × kilimandscharicum*, which is a hybrid between sweet basil and camphor basil, *O. kilimandscharicum*.

The many essential oils in basils mean that the genus has a strong stimulant effect, helping to clear the mind and relieve stress, for who hasn't breathed in a little deeper after tearing up some basil? The stimulant effect is supposed to increase circulation to the brain and improve memory. Basil also helps sore sinuses and soothes headaches. A simple inhalation of basil in hot water will help a tender head feel restored and is said to help with hay fever.

Holy basil, or tulsi, is a sacred herb to the Vaishnava tradition of Hinduism and is also widely used in Ayurvedic medicine as a fresh tea, a dried powder or with its fresh leaf mixed with ghee to treat a number of ailments.

## How to grow

Basil is a herb that loves the sun and will need to be started off indoors, either on a sunny windowsill or in a heated propagator. It germinates between 15–20°C/59–68°F. My best results come from tamping down the compost in a small pot and sowing the seeds on to the surface of the soil, gently pressing into the compost, but not covering them up. Good light assists with quick germination. Likewise, humidity is hugely important in the first few days, and covering the pot with a clear plastic bag or propagator lid will speed up germination, although these should be removed as soon as the first leaves are through to allow air circulation. When the baby plants have their first true leaves (as opposed to the seedling leaves, which are larger and often simpler-looking), prick out into individual pots. Sweet basils can be planted outside, though slugs love them and they don't like temperatures below 10–12°C/50–53°F. Holy basil is far more tender and may need to be grown indoors on a sunny windowsill as it dislikes temperatures below 16°C/60°F. Good light is essential for growth.

## How to use

Once a plant has six to eight pairs of leaves they can be picked. Pinching them out at a leaf node will allow the plant to branch out. The flowers are nice in tea, imparting a sweet, subtle basil flavour. However, if you leave the flowers, you will get seed. This can be used to make the traditional Asian drinks falooda or sabja (basil seed) lemonade, both of which are rich in antioxidants, protein, fibre and essential fats, and are said (though the research is very limited and as of yet inconclusive) to help with controlling blood sugar as well as improving the skin. Take 2 teaspoons of soaked seeds every day. In traditional medicine basil seed is often used to treat colds, flu, coughs and asthma with its antibacterial and antispasmodic properties. It is also thought that the outer coating of the seed may help with stomach cramps and indigestion.

Basil seed should be soaked in a little water, just enough to cover the seeds. After 5 minutes you will see a jelly-like covering, but for the best results soak for an hour when the whole thing will become a thick, gelatinous mixture. The gelatinous seeds are very good in milky drinks, such as coconut or cow's milk. You can also soak the seeds directly in milk rather than water if preferred.

## Holy basil tea

Holy basil tea is wonderful-tasting and aromatic, with strong spicy notes, somewhere between black pepper, sweet basil and mint. It is said to reduce anxiety and is a good drink to try if you are cutting down on coffee because it is energizing without that caffeine hit. You can use either fresh or dried leaves. Start by using 1 teaspoon of dried leaves to 2 cups of water and adjust by taste. I like 2 or 3 fresh leaves per cup that is covered while it brews (so as not to lose the volatile oils).

## Holy basil syrup

A syrup of the fresh leaves of holy basil is known to be good for soothing upper respiratory infections, such as coughs, colds and flu. This can be made with honey, which brings out the unique peppery taste of the herb. Bring ½ cup of water to the boil and steep with either 2 tablespoons of finely cut fresh herbs or 1 tablespoon of dried herb in a heatproof container. Steep for at least 15 minutes, then strain, squeezing to extract as much liquid as possible from the herbs, and then combine with ½ cup of honey. This will store for 2 weeks in the fridge. You can also infuse the herbs directly into the honey, using 2 tablespoons of herbs per cup. Infuse for around 5 days and then strain the honey through a sieve.

# BLACKBERRY,

*see* RASPBERRY

---

# BORAGE

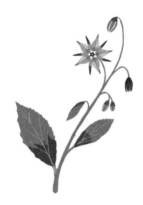

**Other Name** Starflower.

**Botanical Names** *Borago officinalis, Borago officinalis* 'Alba'.

**Family** Boraginaceae.

**Parts Used** Flowers, young leaves, seeds.

**Plant Properties** Relaxant, demulcent, tonic.

**Uses** Anti-inflammatory; good for gastrointestinal issues, such as cramps and colic; and as a mild diuretic. It is often prescribed in natural medicine as a good remedy for PMS. The seed is commercially used as a source of GLA (gamma linoleic acid), a fatty acid that reduces inflammation in the body.

**Preparations** Culinary, including dried flowers; infusions, strewing herb for baths, teas.

**Considerations** While there's a long tradition across the Mediterranean of eating young borage leaves (and I certainly eat my fair share every spring), they do contain small amounts of pyrrolizidine alkaloids, which are toxic to the liver. This can also be present in borage-flower honey. Hepatotoxicity has been reported after prolonged use of concentrated formulas.

**Tinctures and teas should not be used during pregnancy.**

Borage gives courage and good heart. It is said to comfort the weary and give spark to the melancholy. Francis Bacon and John Gerard, an influential sixteenth-century English botanist who wrote a famous herbal, both thought the herb was an effective antidepressant and Gerard recommended the flower in salads 'to drive away of sorrow and increase the joy of the minde'.* In herbal medicine it is often used as a tonic for the over-stressed. Borage flower is a source of fibre and essential fatty acids, and contains B vitamins, which promote better energy. It is also rich in mucilage, so it is said to help soothe the stomach and aid digestion. On top of all this it is a wonderful plant for bees and will be visited all day long by honeybees and bumbles when in flower.

I use borage a lot in the kitchen, particularly the leaves, which I steam and eat much like spinach. I also dry the flowers, often along with calendula petals. Added to dried oats for muesli, they can bring joy to a simple breakfast, and the blue flowers look particularly magnificent in baked goods such as scones.

I also add borage flowers to ice cubes. The flowers have a sweet, honeyed nature and taste strongly of cucumber. They have traditionally been used in Pimm's and other sweet cup drinks, as well as to flavour gins.

The old leaves are very hairy and can cause contact dermatitis, so it's worth wearing gloves if weeding around them. The young leaves are the most tender and bring the same cucumber taste as the flower, along with a fresh, grassy flavour. The very youngest leaves can be eaten raw, but leaves between 5–10cm long should be boiled, steamed or wilted. Borage leaves are used in traditional German green sauce

*John Gerard, *The Herball or Generall Historie of Plantes*, 1st ed. (London: John Norton, 1597).

recipes, which are often eaten with boiled eggs and can be used in soups or to stuff pastas such as ravioli. *Preboggion* is a northern Italian mixture used to stuff pasta of wild leafy greens, often containing borage, chervil and bladder campion, which are found on the Ligurian coast.

# How to grow

Borage is very easy to grow from seed and once you have it in your garden or pots, you'll find it will happily self-seed thanks to all the bees' hard work. Borage will grow in sun or part shade in a wide range of soils, though it slightly prefers free-draining ones. It should be sown outdoors when the daffodils are in flower. You can direct sow in the garden or into small pots or modules. The slugs tend to leave the hairy leaves alone once the plants are big enough but may munch at young plants. I grow rows of borage on the allotment both for the young leaves and for its industrious flower production. I like 'Alba', the pure white form, because it looks so pretty, but without doubt the straight species with their sky-blue flowers are best for drying or drinks.

# How to use

## For culinary use

Borage flowers should be picked fairly early in the morning and dried somewhere warm, away from direct sunlight, perhaps on a clean tea towel for about a day. When ready they'll feel papery to touch and won't roll into a ball. If you wish, you can remove the stamens before drying, to leave just the pretty star-shaped petals. Store in an airtight container out of direct sunlight.

To make pleasing ice cubes add a single flower to each well before you put the tray in the freezer.

The flowers can be added to sun tea (where you use the sun to brew the flavour into water, see page 19) or to flavour water with the delicious taste of cucumber. Likewise, they make a lovely addition to summer salads.

The leaves can be used to make a nice after-dinner drink to aid digestion. Use 1 teaspoon of dried leaves per cup, and limit to 1 cup a day because the leaves are known to contain alkaloids (see Considerations). Alternatively, if wilting the leaves, drink the remaining water. Borage tea tastes best with lemon verbena, lemon balm or a lemon slice added for a little flavour.

## For medicinal use

Traditionally the young leaves have been used to make a poultice to draw out infection and reduce swelling; the leaves were mashed up before applying to the affected area. I have little experience of using borage leaves to reduce swelling, but have used comfrey leaves (in the same family) for years to reduce swollen ankles and minor sprains. I suggest wrapping the area with thin gauze, applying the mash and then covering with more gauze or lint. Leave the mash on until it starts to turn black, remove and compost, and reapply with fresh mash. For sprains I tend to try to do at least 24 hours with a poultice.

# BUGLE

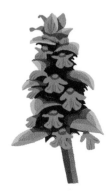

**Other Names** Bugleweed, blue bugle, common bugle.

**Botanical Name** *Ajuga reptans.*

**Family** Lamiaceae (mint family).

**Parts Used** All aerial parts, leaves, stems, flowers.

**Plant Properties** Anti-inflammatory, pain-relieving.

**Uses** Externally for wounds, cuts, ulcers and insect bites.

**Preparations** Decoctions, poultices, teas.

**Considerations** None known.

Other than nibbling at hawthorn leaves for a good heart and rubbing dock on to nettle rash, bugle was my first foray into plant medicine. My lovely assistant head gardener, Joe, had a cut on his thumb from a pruning saw. Being on his knuckle, it was ragged and raw, and refused to mend. As we sat drinking our tea I made a simple poultice from the bugle growing in the lawn and made him promise that he would leave it on overnight. The next day the cut had knitted together and its angry redness reduced. I think we were both a little shocked at how quickly this 'carpenter's plant' worked.

But bugle has a long and wide history across the Mediterranean of being a 'woundwort' of a plant, often used to stem bleeding and heal ugly cuts. Clearly if you chopped your leg off, I wouldn't hand you a poultice of leaves, but for scrapes, cuts and insect bites when you might resort to a regular plaster, bugle is your go-to; you can even stick the leaves underneath the plaster. Traditionally poultices were made by chewing the herb and spitting the mulch on to the wound. After all, out in the woods, your mouth might be a great deal more sterile than the other options available.

## How to grow

*Ajuga reptans* is a wild weed of lawns and grassy spots, particularly of rich, damp soils in sun or part shade. There are numerous cultivars bred for the garden because it makes an excellent ground-cover plant, spreading into a tight carpet of evergreen leaves that doesn't mind gentle footfall, and the flowers are much loved by bees. It needs little or no attention; you can cut off the flowers after they have finished if you want, but other than that bugle is happy to get on with things by itself. Catlin's Giant is a supersized version with flower spikes up to 30–45cm high, covered in those lovely purple flowers. There is also a popular dark purple variety called 'Atropurpurea' and another dark bronzed one called 'Braunherz' that both look particularly arresting as ground cover under trees.

# How to use

## For culinary use

You can make a basic tea or decoction using either fresh or dried herbs (see page 18). This tea is said to be good for coughs, sprains, bruising and tendonitis, and many believe that taking this herb internally as well as externally helps speed healing. Drink 2–3 cups a day. The decoction can also be soaked into bandages and applied to the affected area.

You can also infuse leaves, flowers and stems in oil (jojoba or olive oil) using the herbal oil method (see page 25). This oil can be used in place of decoction and is very good for bruises.

## For medicinal use

A poultice of leaves, stems and flowers can be easily mashed using a clean pestle and mortar. Richo Cech, in *Making Plant Medicines*, writes charmingly that you should 'worry the fresh leaves until juice extrudes, then plaster to the affected area'. A plaster or micropore tape will help to retain the plant's precious juices.

# CAMOMILE

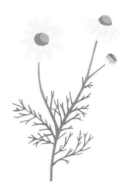

**Botanical Name** *Matricaria recutita* (*M. chamomilla* is a common misnomer. Not to be confused with Roman camomile, *Chamaemelum nobile*.)

**Family** Asteraceae (sunflower or daisy family).

**Parts Used** Flowers.

**Plant Properties** Relaxant, carminative, anti-inflammatory, antispasmodic.

**Uses** Insomnia, anxiety, indigestion, diarrhoea, colic, flu, migraines, teething, motion sickness, burns, rashes or otherwise inflamed skin.

**Preparations** Poultices, strewing herb for baths, teas.

**Considerations** Some people get a headache if they drink too much of this tea; if you find yourself experiencing this, camomile tea is not for you. Avoid if you have a known allergy to the Asteraceae family.

Gentle camomile to send you and Peter Rabbit softly off to sleep, to calm a worried head in the middle of the night, to soothe and settle an upset stomach before bed. Read about camomile in any herbal and the list of its capabilities will be long: from soothing conjunctivitis to dealing with neuralgia. For most people a cup or two of camomile is all they need before they can barely keep their eyes open. It doesn't actually send you to sleep – it's not a sedative – but it does relax you to a point where sleep is the best option. To best describe a plant as gentle seems a bit feeble, but the truth is that is what camomile does best: calms and cools. It does have a bitter flavour, but far less pronounced than shop-bought stuff. I marry it with sweet oat stems, lavender, lime blossom and other gentle herbs for a bedtime tea.

Alongside aloe, camomile is my go-to remedy for sunburnt skin. A cool camomile tea or a bath strewn with the flower heads are my favourite ways to reduce the heat and pain. I've read that it makes an excellent bath for sleep-deprived children or those who are teething. Indeed, camomile's anti-inflammatory properties, both internally and externally, are well documented. The tea is said to be effective for respiratory and digestive systems and helps prevent stomach ulcers. It is a mild antimicrobial, worth taking if you have a cold or the flu, and is said to be helpful against the symptoms of hay fever. You can take in inhalation either with the essential oil or with a strong tea to relieve irritated sinuses. One study also found camomile to be as beneficial as a chlorhexidine mouthwash for gingivitis.*

## How to grow

The fabled camomile lawn with its sweet apple scent is actually the Roman camomile, *Chamaemelum nobile*, rather than the versatile German camomile, which grows to 60cm high and so forms more

* Forêt, R. D. L., *The Alchemy of Herbs: Transform Everyday Ingredients into Foods and Remedies That Heal,* 1st ed. (Carlsbad, California: Hay House, Inc., 2017).

of a bush than a lawn. Originally from southern Europe, it's now naturalized in the UK and is often found growing as an arable weed. Camomile grows best in free-draining soil; it doesn't need particularly rich soil to do well. It must be grown in full sun. It can be successfully incorporated into a garden border, and is perhaps best grown near the front as it's fairly short and somewhat floppy. It can be grown in a pot, though it may need some sort of support, such as a pea stick.

German camomile germinates between 15–20°C /59–68°F and should be sown in spring, directly into the ground once the soil has warmed up. If you sow earlier, you will need to do so indoors. As the seed is very fine it can often get lost, so I prefer to sow in seed trays, pricking out once the seedlings are large enough to handle. Do not cover the seed with compost; light aids germination.

Harvest the flowers when they are fully open. High temperatures can destroy the plant's volatile oils, so dry the flowers somewhere cool, away from direct sunlight. Place them on a plate rather than hanging upside down as they tend to crumble. Don't worry if the flower heads fall apart or if they've already lost their ray petals; the immature seed makes an equally good tea. The more you pick, the more the plants will flower; therefore you may end up picking small handfuls every other day rather than having one big harvest. Once dried, store in an airtight jar away from a heat source or direct sun.

# How to use

## Camomile tea

You can use small amounts of dried camomile flowers and steep quickly to make a delicate tisane. For a stronger tea brew 1 teaspoon of flower heads in 1 cup of boiling water for 10 minutes in a covered container. This can be drunk three or four times a day.

Add equal parts fennel seed for a more palatable tea. Fennel also aids digestion, is anti-inflammatory and boosts circulation.

If you are growing your own flowers, try the tea with fresh flower heads. It has a very different taste, slightly sweet and more perfumed.

For the perfect bedtime treat combine 1 teaspoon of dried camomile, 2 teaspoons of dried oat straw, 2 teaspoons of rose petals, ½ teaspoon of lavender flowers and ½ teaspoon of lemon balm. Steep the herbs in a teapot for at least 10 minutes, strain, and add honey if desired.

## For medicinal use

Dried camomile flowers can also be added to bath salts to make a relaxing pre-bedtime soak.

Camomile can be used as a poultice: make up a strong tea and soak a clean cotton bandage in the liquid. Add 2 cups of strong tea to a basin of water with Epsom salts added to make an antibacterial soak for sore feet.

For an eye wash for tired eyes, use a mixture of salt and dried flower heads and distilled water. Add ½ teaspoon sea salt and 2 teaspoons of camomile per cup of water that has been boiled and allowed to cool until warm. Use in an eye bath. This mixture should not be stored and the eye bath and all instruments used to make the wash need to be sterile, so boil them before use. Alternatively use a teabag of dried camomile or wrap dried camomile flowers in a clean muslin, soften in hot water, then allow to cool and place this on your eyes.

A strong brew of camomile can also be rinsed through hair after shampooing as a rinse to lighten. This works best on blonde hair and has the extra bonus of making it feel lovely and soft.

# CARAWAY

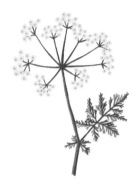

**Botanical Name** *Carum carvi.*
**Family** Apiaceae (carrot family).
**Parts Used** Seeds.
**Plant Properties** Carminative, antispasmodic, expectorant, astringent, antimicrobial.
**Uses** Digestion; to ease flatulence and colic; to stimulate appetite; as a treatment for diarrhoea with antispasmodic actions; can help relieve menstrual cramp.
**Preparations** Teas.
**Considerations** None known.

Caraway, that clean flavour with a hint of liquorice so perfect in good bread or a buttery biscuit, is also a gentle and calming herb to our insides. Safe for children, a simple tea made by steeping seeds in hot water will ease upset or colicky stomachs, calm the spasms that come with diarrhoea and can even help with period pains. It's pretty delicious too, so it's no hardship to drink. It is also said that gargling this liquid can be a great help with laryngitis.

# How to grow

Caraway is a biennial, so it flowers and fruits in its second year. It has a very pretty umbel flower head, whose frothy white flowers grow in midsummer above fern-like foliage. It can be found wild growing in meadows and prefers full sun, in rich but well-drained soil. It can, however, do perfectly well in semi-shade. It looks much like cow parsley only smaller, and grows well in containers (make sure you use deep pots of 30cm or more to accommodate the taproots) or in the garden among other flowers. Two or three plants will give you plenty of seeds for the next year. Like all members of the Apiaceae family the seed is best sown fresh, otherwise it can be slow to germinate. Young year-old plants are easy enough to source from garden centres ready to flower. Seed should be harvested when the flower head is brown and the seeds completely dry. If wet weather prevents this, cut the whole seed head off and hang upside down in a paper bag somewhere warm and dry.

# How to use

### Caraway tea

A simple tea can be drunk up to three times a day. To make an infusion pour 1 cup of boiling water over 1 teaspoon of crushed seeds (use a pestle and mortar) and allow to steep in a covered container for 10–15 minutes.

# CHERVIL

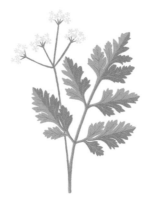

**Other Names**  French parsley, garden chervil.

**Botanical Name**  *Anthriscus cerefolium*.

**Family**  Apiaceae (carrot family).

**Parts Used**  Aerial parts.

**Plant Properties**  Mild stimulant, improves digestion, expectorant, diuretic.

**Uses**  Eye wash, wound-healing, improves digestion, spring tonic.

**Preparations**  Culinary, poultices.

**Considerations**  Can cause contact dermatitis in some individuals.

I have dug under snow to find a few of chervil's fine filigree leaves to add to a soup or salad. It has a flavour suggestive of aniseed and is one of the '*fines herbes*' of a bouquet garni in French cuisine. Its delicate flavour is suited to white fish, omelettes, goat's cheese and other mild, soft cheeses. Pick a few of its flowers in spring for seasoning, but do so sparingly for not only will they provide you with seed for the next year's sowing, they will also please the bees and hoverflies.

Chervil is not often used medicinally, but it does make a good spring tonic for cleansing the liver and kidneys and settling the digestion. It's certainly one herb that is in ready supply before it flowers and I eat it in salads all spring. The bruised raw leaves can be used as a poultice for slow-healing wounds and it is said that you can make an eye wash out of the leaves to treat inflamed eyes.

## How to grow

Chervil is a winter herb so it's best to germinate in the warm soils of late summer and grow into the cool season. Start chervil off in the place in which it is to grow. Its long taproot means it dislikes transplanting and doing so can trigger it to rapidly bolt. Sow somewhere cool and moist; I like to grow mine by the edge of the path so that it's easy to reach in winter. It grows to around 30–60cm tall when in flower. Sow any time from March to August 1cm deep and cover with a little soil. Early-spring sowings often result in the plant flowering early, leaving few leaves. Seedlings can be slow to germinate and take up to three weeks to appear. Chervil is a prolific self-seeder and if they like you, they can take over. However, I find that chervil is adored by slugs (such gourmands!) and most of my seedlings get mown down by them, so I end up with a good balance of nicely scattered plants without having to do much weeding.

The young leaves should be ready to harvest around nine weeks after sowing. You can make several cuts and it will respond with new leaves, until the plant starts to flower and the leaves become coarser and less flavoursome.

# CHICKWEED

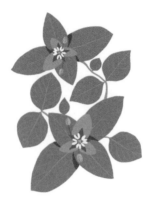

**Botanical Name** *Stellaria media.*
**Family** Caryophyllaceae
(pink family).
**Parts Used** Entire plant, but mostly
stems, leaves and flowers. Must be
harvested when young and fresh
in autumn and late winter or early
spring.
**Plant Properties** Nutritive, emollient,
relieves inflammations and
irritations.

**Uses** An external remedy for
cuts, minor wounds,
inflammation and itching.
Very nutritious.
**Preparations** Culinary, infused
water, poultices, strewing herb for
baths, teas.
**Considerations** Eating large
amounts will act as a mild
laxative.

*Stellaria* means 'little stars', referring to the tiny white flowers of this wayside weed. Chickweed loves to grow in damp grass, in the cracks in paths and along pavements, in rich pastures, and in the vegetable garden. When it is fat and healthy it's such a good green for eating: sweet and slightly nutty. It is a highly nutritious green, being rich in vitamin C, A and B complexes, as well as a good source for minerals such as calcium, magnesium, manganese, zinc, iron and phosphorus. It's a favourite foraged food for early spring. Fair warning: a fat, healthy plant on the edge of a pavement has probably thrived there because of dog pee.

Chickweed is a seasonal herb and does not do well dried, so use it fresh. I love to add it to green sauces and salsas, to chop it into salads or to make a pesto. It can also be added to smoothies. You can cook it, but you lose much of its nutritious value and it tastes so good raw that it seems a waste to wilt it away. Still, it's a very good vehicle for butter.

The name 'chickweed' comes from its long use for feeding to hens to increase egg size and improve overall production and the nutritional value of the eggs, particularly in the good omega-3s and -6s. Chickweed contains saponins – these are chemical substances found in the plant that foam when added to water, which is detectable in the slightly soapy taste when you eat the leaves. These saponins are said to help remove toxins from the gastrointestinal system and for that reason it is often referred to as a 'spring-cleanse' herb.

In herbal medicine chickweed is famed for its ability to ease skin complaints and relieve itching. I like to add handfuls of the herb to the bath to soothe my dry and itchy skin.

## How to grow

Honestly I'm not even sure you could get seeds of this weed. You probably have plenty already, so forage for it on good clean ground. You don't have to grow it; it will come to you, but you do need to learn to notice where it does best in your garden so that you can harvest succulent leaves. It likes cool, damp, slightly shaded spots, and often does well growing up a wall. If you harvest it all without letting a little go to seed, you'll have missed your next window of free plants.

# How to use

Chickweed is said to mildly suppress your appetite and therefore can be used as a weight-loss aid. Make an infusion to drink before meals. Pour 1 cup of boiling water over 200g of chickweed and drink up to three times a day. This infusion can also be used as an eye wash to soothe irritated eyes. Make daily.

## For medicinal use
To make a poultice mash the stems, leaves and flowers so that juices flow and apply to the wound, cut or irritated skin using a soft bandage.

# CHILLI

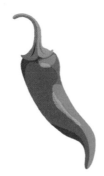

**Other Names** Cayenne pepper, chilli pepper, pepper.

**Botanical Name** *Capsicum* species.

**Family** Solanaceae (nightshade family).

**Parts Used** Fruit.

**Plant Properties** Stimulant, carminative, antimicrobial, antifungal, stimulates blood flow, particularly to the skin.

**Uses** To ward off colds; to stimulate blood flow in poor circulation; to help against chilblains; as a mild anaesthetic for nerve and muscle pain, such as toothache.

**Preparations** Culinary, salves, teas.

**Considerations** Although there are no known side effects to taking chillis, as anyone who's not washed their hands properly after preparing a chilli for cooking will know, the fruit, and in particular the seeds, needs to be handled with caution. Get chilli into your eyes and it can be truly painful; wash out with water or milk. Wear goggles and ventilate the room well when grinding pepper. Even drying peppers in a dehydrator will fill the house with a burning heat if you're not careful. After use, wash down any tools or machinery with alcohol, then soap and then water to remove all traces.

I f the fire and burn of the chilli fruit has you reaching for the hot sauce to add to almost anything and the sweat from a spicy meal is your idea of satisfaction, then your body already knows the good that cayenne pepper can do for you. Chilli is a good digestive stimulant and peppers the dullest of foods so that, for a devotee, a meal without is just bland. Many will also have used Tiger balms or other salves for muscle ache that contain a concentration of dried chilli or extract to relieve tired or strained muscles, but less well known is the sweating away of the first hint of a cold with chilli tea. However, many people have a constitution that just doesn't cope well with the heat. No matter how effective chilli remedies may be, if your idea of hell is hot spice, then you shouldn't go near them. Herbalists often describe people who love chillies as being cool or of cool constitution; they might have cold hands and sluggish digestion, so the heat of chilli provides a kick to their circulatory system.

Chillies range in heat from the mild and fruity to the frankly impossible. Their effect is measured using Scoville heat units: a sweet pepper has 0 SHU, a mild cayenne 30,000 and a Scotch bonnet over 100,000. The hottest chilli to date is the Carolina Reaper, which comes in at 2,200,000. I'm not sure it's even humanly possible to eat that, though I am sure plenty of daredevils have tried. There are lots of hot chillies out there, but those that don't bite too hard are far more enjoyable to cook with. Chillies originate from South and Central America but are now widespread around the world. They were cultivated as long as 6000 years ago by people in the Americas and were introduced to the rest of the world after the Columbian exchange, a widespread transfer of plants, animals, culture and human populations between the Americas and the Old World in the fifteenth and sixteenth centuries.

Chilli has long been used in folk medicine to promote a healthy heart and this seems to be beginning to be backed up by science. There have been numerous conflicting studies on cayenne and its potential medicinal outcomes; however, some of these have shown it to have positive results for digestion, if taken regularly, and recent findings have shown that cayenne potentially has a protective effect on the stomach.* Studies have also shown that regular chilli consumption results in a decreased resting heart rate.

Likewise, herbalist and folk medicine has long promoted chilli for chilblains and cold feet and hands. Rubbing chilli into the chest to relieve chest infections will certainly increase blood flow to the skin and this will alleviate certain symptoms. Chilli is even a famed diet weapon: we're told, eat plenty and your metabolism will speed up. But it's not a miracle fix. Chocolate chilli cake is still cake.

## How to grow

The chilli gang is broad and diverse. It ranges from the popular *Capsicum annuum*, an annual that encompasses sweet peppers, jalapeños and common cayenne to Bolivian species that grow high in the mountains – short-lived perennials that reach up to 2 metres tall and don't mind cooler weather. Bolivia is still a lot warmer and sunnier than my bit of the world, and if you want to grow chillies at home, it's wise to start them off very early in the year.

Chillies are the first thing that I sow in late winter. A week after New Year's, when the gloom of January starts to loom large, I jolly

* Forêt, R. D. L., *Alchemy of Herbs*, p. 270.

myself with rows of chilli seeds. I grow a huge range of varieties, from outdoor types for damp English summers to specialist Thai chillies that I have to cajole into life with my warmest windowsill or a space in my polytunnel. Many seed packets suggest you can wait till March to sow, but my experience is that if you can grow the plants to a decent size by April, then you've got a good chance of fruit whatever the weather throws at you.

Chillies need to be germinated at a temperature between 15–25°C/ 59–77°F and can be slow to germinate if the soil dries out. I tend to use a propagator lid or a clear plastic bag over 9cm pots. The trick with chillies is to understand how hungry they are. When you see roots poking out of the bottom of the pot you need to pot up to the next size container. Repotting may be a bit of a faff, but providing a new source of compost for the roots to explore results in steady, strong growth, which in turn promotes flowering. You can grow chillies outside in the garden; my limited experiments show that these fruits are much hotter than those grown in pots, but a wet summer will wipe out your harvest. These days I grow some plants in pots on my sunny patio and the rest either on a windowsill or in the polytunnel.

Often you'll find that the first chilli to form is the king chilli, which is in the axis of the first branching stems. It's called the king chilli because if left in place it will rob all the future chillies of nutrients, so it certainly pays to remove this one, otherwise you can end up with one big chilli that's hogging all the energy. Pinch out the growing tips of your chillies to get them to branch out, which will also promote more flowering. I tend to do this around May, when the plants are moving into their final pot. When flowers appear start regularly feeding with an organic liquid fertilizer, such as comfrey or seaweed.

# How to use

You can use a therapeutic dose of 1–5g of powdered cayenne a day. Start on a low dose and work up slowly.

## Chilli tea for colds

When you feel that first tickle in your throat make a cup of chilli tea. It is said to speed up the healing process and shorten the duration of the cold, and it will also soothe an irritated throat.

Powdered cayenne is best, but you can use dried instead as long as you strain out the seed – getting one stuck in your throat is not fun.

Bring 1 cup of water to the boil. Place ¼ teaspoon of cayenne and ½ teaspoon of crushed chilli in a cup, and pour over the water. Allow to steep for 5–10 minutes. Add lemon juice, honey and/or a little cinnamon to taste. Slowly sip the tea while it is still hot and prepare to sweat out that cold. This can be drunk up to three times a day.

## Fermented chilli sauce

I love this fermented sauce; it's very easy to make, and can be adapted easily. You can blend together mild and hot chillies, add garlic and onions if you wish, and make it as thick or thin as you please. It will store in the fridge for 3 months.

Take 30 fresh chillies around 5–8cm long, more if you are using small ones. Use ripe red fruits or experiment with green, which will make the sauce taste more sour. If you want a milder sauce, remove the seeds first.

Wearing goggles (the swimming sort will be fine), use a food blender to mash up the chillies, then stir in 1 teaspoon of sea salt. At this stage you can also add a clove or two of crushed garlic or a small minced onion. I've heard of grated carrot being added to sweeten it too.

Using a rubber-sealed preserving jar or a clear glass jar with fitted lid, press down the mixture in the jar, place the lid on and leave overnight. Check the mixture the next day. If there's no liquid around the mash, you may need to add another pinch of salt or a salt solution of one to four parts water. Leave the mixture at room temperature and stir once a week. You may well see a soft white bloom of mould, which is nothing to worry about. Mix this in and it will disappear (some people swear this mould adds to the flavour). However, a blue, green or black mould should be skimmed off. Once removed shake a little more salt on the mixture to prevent further mould. I like to leave this hot sauce to ferment for at least 6 weeks, though I left one batch of very hot chillies to ferment for 3 months and I was impressed with the flavour.

You can use this chilli mash as a condiment. I don't recommend cooking with it because heat destroys all the good bacteria developed during the fermenting process. Alternatively use cider vinegar to dilute the chilli mash into something closer to sauce. The quantity of cider vinegar required will vary from batch to batch. I add 1 tablespoon at a time until I achieve the desired consistency and flavour; it's up to you what that is, but something that is runny enough to come out of a bottle is wise. You can then strain out the seeds and pulp to get a Tabasco-like sauce, or leave them in. Often the cider vinegar and mash will separate, so you'll need a container that will allow you to shake it before using.

# CLEAVERS

**Other Names** Sticky willy, sticky weed, sticky jack, sticky bud, stickeljack, grip grass, goosegrass.

**Botanical Name** *Galium aparine.*

**Family** Rubiaceae (madder family).

**Parts Used** Stems, leaves.

**Plant Properties** Diuretic, kidney tonic, lymphatic, anti-inflammatory, tonic, astringent.

**Uses** Spring tonic to stimulate lymphatic system; poultices for skin inflammations.

**Preparations** Culinary, infusions, smoothies, teas.

**Considerations** Some people suffer from contact dermatitis when handling the raw stems.

Cleavers, or sticky willy, is a wonderful wayside plant of hedgerows and banks, which when plucked and thrown at your opponent will stick to their hair or clothes. Generally it is best thrown on the opponent's back to turn them into a walking hedgerow without their knowledge. The barb hooks are there to help the plant to scramble up hedgerows and to distribute seed. Dogs, sheep, goats and the like then move this plant to new ground. Its other name is goosegrass, so called because geese truly do love to eat it. The young stems when still tender make a good green, particularly as a vehicle for butter and salt.

Cleavers are a spring green. By May they become too tough to eat; the barbed hooks that make it so good for throwing at people make the stems distinctly prickly to eat once grown. Tender cleaver leaves appear in the hungry gap when the garden isn't offering much and have traditionally been used as a spring tonic. You can juice them or infuse handfuls in water for 24 hours to make a tea from the leaves, which, it is said, is one of the best tonics available for the lymphatic system. It is reported to be helpful with adenoids and tonsillitis. A poultice of mashed stems and leaves is also said to help with skin irritations.

## How to grow

You don't have to grow this one; it is a wild thing, so ubiquitous that any park or disused plot will have plenty growing, but like all wild things it needs to come from clean ground, not near roads or industrial sites. It will appear in most gardens and allotments and particularly likes disturbed ground. Harvest in spring when the stems and leaves are supple and bright green.

## How to use

It's hard to dry cleavers thoroughly because the plant has a high water content and therefore I consider this as a very seasonal herb, ready when you need to shift from winter to spring. If you do want to dry it, then you'll need a screen to harvest very gently, ensuring you don't crush the stems. Turn frequently and provide some sort of airflow or gentle heat, perhaps over a radiator.

Hot water destroys the most nutritious part of cleavers, so if you are making a tea, use warm water. Alternatively mash or juice the stems and freeze them in ice cubes for future use. They will store for a couple of months before freezer burn sets in.

## Cleavers water

Take a large handful of the stems and leaves and infuse in 1 litre of water for 6–12 hours. Add lemon and ginger or cucumber for a more refreshing drink (see page 19). Drink within 24 hours, before the water starts to ferment.

# CORIANDER

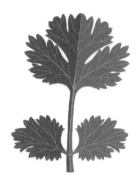

**Other Name** Cilantro.

**Botanical Name** *Coriandrum sativum.*

**Family** Apiaceae (carrot family).

**Parts Used** Fresh leaves, stems, green seeds, dried seeds, roots.

**Plant Properties** Carminative, improves digestion.

**Uses** To aid digestion, to relieve cramps and griping from wind and gas.

**Preparations** Culinary, teas.

**Considerations** Some people show allergies to the Apiaceae family.

Coriander is such a popular culinary herb. It has a wide geographical distribution, spanning from southern Europe to northern Africa and south-western Asia, which accounts for its popularity in so many cuisines. It is thought that it originally came from Iran and it has had a long history of cultivation. About half a pint of coriander seed was found in Tutankhamen's tomb and as it was not a wild plant in Egypt archaeologists have concluded it must have been cultivated by ancient Egyptians. Coriander is often associated with South American, particularly Mexican, cuisine, but actually it was rather a late introduction and only appeared there around the seventeenth century. However, other herbs used in Mexican cuisine, such as culantro, quinquilla or papalo, have similar flavour profiles, and coriander is most likely now a substitute for these.

Coriander has a distinct flavour and is a wonderful addition to many dishes, at least to those who love it. To these people it is grassy, with a lemon- or lime-like flavour, fresh with woody notes. It tempers well to saltiness, deodorizes fishiness and cools hot, spicy food. Those who hate it will declare that it tastes of soap and something rotten. The camp you fall into will apparently depend on genetic preference; some people are just born disliking this herb.

Some people are allergic to coriander. It belongs to the Apiaceae family, along with carrots and parsnips. This family is known to cause food allergies in a small percentage of the population. For the rest of us, though, coriander is an incredibly nutritious herb. The stems and leaves are rich in vitamins A, C and K, with moderate amounts of dietary minerals. The fresh and dried seed has fewer vitamins, but significant amounts of dietary fibre, calcium, selenium, iron, magnesium and manganese. In herbalism the leaf, stem and fresh green seeds are all known to have a particularly good effect on the digestive tract, dispelling gas and combating flatulence. This perhaps is one reason why coriander leaf goes so well with bean dishes. The root is also edible and has a strong, slightly sweeter flavour that is quite delicious. It's used in widely in Thai dishes and soups.

# How to grow

Coriander is very easy to grow. It's a cool-climate crop, so can successfully grow all winter long with a little protection. In hotter months it will want to bolt, then you'll lose leaf production but it will soon flower, with fresh seed following. Sow coriander in pots or direct in the ground from mid-spring onwards. I like to scatter handfuls of seed around the garden because the flowers attract so many beneficial insects, in particular hoverflies, the larvae of which eat up to 150 aphids a day before they mature into flies.

# How to use

Eat as much leaf as pleases you for its vitamin-rich properties. The seed is used as a carminative and digestive aid and can be mixed with honey and eaten before a meal. Use ½ teaspoon of fresh seeds with 1 teaspoon of honey or make it into a tea. It's not unpleasant tea, but a little strange. For a more pleasant beverage you can mix it with aniseed, fennel, celery and cardamom for a clean digestive tea.

## Coriander tea for digestion

1–2 teaspoons whole dried fennel seed
½ teaspoon whole dried coriander seed
½ teaspoon aniseed seed
¼ teaspoon celery seed
3 cups water
Fresh ginger (optional)
Honey (optional)

Coarsely grind the seed in a coffee grinder or pestle and mortar to create a powder. Bring 3 cups of water to the boil and stir in the powder. Simmer for 5 minutes, covering the saucepan. Allow the mixture to steep for another 10 minutes in a covered container, then strain and serve. Add fresh ginger and honey to taste. This tea is very refreshing when allowed to cool and served over ice.

# DANDELION

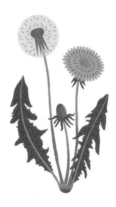

**Botanical Name** *Taraxicum officinale.*
**Family** Asteraceae (sunflower or daisy family).
**Parts Used** Flowers, leaves, roots.
**Plant Properties** Bitter, improves digestion, diuretic.

**Uses** Digestive tonic for the urinary system; often used as a diuretic to aid kidney functions.
**Preparations** Culinary, coffee substitute, infusions.
**Considerations** None known.

In May and June when every bank is covered with brilliant bright yellow discs of gold between globes of fluffy seed heads, it seems extraordinary to me that we wage a war on these plants. Not only is it a cheeringly pretty plant; in removing it we are desperately trying to eliminate such a helpful medicine. Dandelions have been used for centuries as a diuretic and this is reflected in their French common name *pissenlit* (*piss en lit*), meaning 'to wet the bed'. This is not a tea to have before going to sleep. The diuretic properties mean that it aids the kidneys. The root is also used to stimulate bile flow and aid the liver. The root can be dried and used in tea or roasted; prepare as you might a thin parsnip. You can either eat the roots for tea, or chop them up or grind them to use in hot drinks. Traditionally dandelion root has been used with chicory as a coffee substitute, partly because it tastes quite bitter like coffee. I recommend it simmered slowly in oat or nut milk and with just a touch of honey to sweeten. Dandelion leaf can also be combined in equal parts with nettles as a spring tonic.

Every part of the dandelion is good for you and is an excellent tonic for digestion. Eating dandelion root before a meal is said to help increase stomach acid, which in turn helps you to digest your food. If you have a sluggish digestion, then adding dandelion leaves to your salad might help.

## How to grow

Dandelion is a wild weed that is no doubt already growing very happily in your garden. There is a great deal of difference between those that are mowed regularly and grow as flat as a pancake to those that grow in lush long grass. The best roots always come from those that grow in damp, rich soil. If you find all your dandelions are a little thin and tough, you can dig them up to grow in a pot. This may seem like madness, but growing this way will result in thick roots and soft, tender leaves for salads. You can also blanch the leaves as you would endives, by excluding light so they grow pale and sweet. I'm not sure blanching the leaves exactly adds to their medicinal properties, but it makes them taste sweet.

The genus *Taraxicum* has about fifty different species and there are around four distinct cultivars of *T. officinale*. I grow the Asian *T. pseudoroseum*, which has lovely pink flowers and can be used in much the same way as the common dandelion. A garden full of pink dandelions is quite something. There's a French cultivar of *T. officinale* that is sold as 'thick-leaved' or 'Sativum', which has broader leaves that form a clump rather than a rosette and therefore produces more leaf mass, which is good for salads. *T. mongolicum*, the Chinese dandelion also known as pu gong ying, is used in traditional Chinese medicine to eliminate toxins.

For obvious reasons make sure you pick dandelions that haven't been sprayed, aren't near polluted roads or, worse still, grow in an area frequented by dogs.

# How to use

## Dandelion tea

A basic tea of fresh or dried leaves and flowers, up to 200g, can be drunk up to three times a day (but you will go to the loo a lot!). Or try 200g of fresh or dried root three times a day. You can add honey to either tea to make them more palatable.

## Dandelion iced tea

Use either cooled boiled water or the sun tea method (see page 19). Place several handfuls of flowers in a 2-litre jar, add peppermint, lemon balm or lemon verbena for flavour, and let it seep for 30 minutes if using hot water, several hours if using the sun. Make sure to cover the jar when seeping. Strain the flowers out and serve over ice and with honey to sweeten.

## For culinary use

I love to eat the heart of the plant: just 2.5cm or so of the root, peeled with a crown of unopened flower heads and the nubs of the leaves.

The whole thing may just be the size of your thumbnail, but collect enough and sautéed in olive oil and a little salt and served on pasta it makes quite the dish. The leaves are bitter, like a wild-tasting endive, and need to be picked young to be at their most palatable. Their bitterness is where all their health lies and one of the simplest ways to get your dose is to eat the young leaves. There is rarely a point in the year when you can't pick young dandelion leaves, even in deepest winter. They work well when matched with something oily and acidic to cut through the bitterness. A simple salad of mackerel, salad potatoes, minced red onion and young dandelion leaves is a perfect example.

The flower heads, when opened, can be dipped in batter and fried. They can also be steeped in brandy for a digestive tonic. You'll find numerous recipes for dandelion flower wine in other herbals and online.

## Dandelion flower vinegar

This is an easy way to use dandelion flowers and makes a great salad dressing that has plenty of benefits for digestion. You can also make dandelion root vinegar the same way.

Place the dandelions in a wide-necked jar to the top (you'll need about 30–60 flower heads) and cover with apple cider vinegar. Screw the top on tightly. If you are using a jar with a metal top, place a piece of baking parchment between the jar and the lid so that the vinegar doesn't react with the lid. Leave for a month in a dark place and then strain.

# DILL

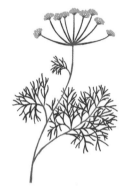

**Other Name** Dill weed.

**Botanical Name** *Anethum graveolens.*

**Family** Apiaceae (carrot family).

**Parts Used** Leaves, seeds, flowers.

**Plant Properties** Stimulates digestion, antispasmodic, carminative, nutritive, antimicrobial, antibacterial.

**Uses** To relieve gas and bloating, treat colic, improve bad breath, improve appetite and aid digestion, relieve piles.

**Preparations** Culinary, teas.

**Considerations** None known.

Dill may take its name from the Norse *dilla*, meaning 'lull', as it is said to have a relaxing effect on the muscles. Dill is well established for the use of relieving stomach cramps, dispelling gas and flatulence and treating colic. Traditionally dill is taken by the mother and passed through her milk to the baby and, in this way, is safe enough to be consumed by children. The seed may be ground up or bruised before making tea. Extract of dill seed has antimicrobial and antibacterial properties and it is said that the tea can also treat urinary infections and help relieve piles.

It's interesting to note how prominent dill is in fermented food. Dill cucumber pickles are the most obvious example, but it can also be found in pickled gravlax, seafood recipes and various central and eastern European fermented milk drinks, such as curds, kefir, yoghurt and buttermilk. This is partly because the sharp flavour combines well with sour ingredients, and one can't help but think that such nourishing traditions must have also recognized that dill's antimicrobial properties help these ferments stay good. Dill also works particularly well with fish and creamy dishes, to say little of how lovely good potatoes are covered in dill and olive oil.

Dill weed, or the leaf, may also be used as a tea, but it's such a delicious herb that it seems to me to make more sense just to eat it. It is high in vitamins A and C, and calcium. The feathery leaves are very good in salads, particularly combined with cucumber: a perfect marriage of cool and clear flavourings. Dill is a complex flavour that starts sweet before anise notes take hold. Eating it during or after a meal may help relieve a full stomach. Supposedly Russian cosmonauts on spaceflights with confined quarters and a closed air supply asked for dill.

## How to grow

Dill is an easy annual to grow, sown in late spring either direct or in pots. Its delicious nature makes it easy slug fodder and young plants can be mown down overnight, particularly in damp weather. For this reason, especially during the beginning of the season, start dill off in small pots or modules and plant out once a good root system has evolved. However, I can't remember the last time I sowed dill as I find it comes up every year in my polytunnel with no effort on my part other than letting a few plants set seed. Although it is possible to grow dill in semi-shade, it grows best in full sun where it will produce more leaves and flowers. Like all plants in the Apiaceae family, the seed is best sown fresh, so save some of your own in an airtight container. After a year or two viability drastically reduces and germination even with fresh seed can be erratic, so be generous. Even in good years I've never thought 'I've got too much dill here.' You can thin plants to 10–15cm apart in each direction.

Dill's feathery leaves can be dried, but most of the punch is dulled during this process. It's possible to freeze the leaves for a cleaner, stronger flavour. The seed is very fragile once ripe and can shatter easily, so monitor your plants and as they start to turn a dull brown collect the seed heads and continue drying indoors if necessary. The acid-yellow flowers make a fine addition to any garden and will attract a host of pollinating insects, in particular hoverflies. Try using the flower heads in pickling and fermenting, where they add a sweet, subtle flavour.

There are numerous cultivars of dill. 'Dutch Mammoth' dill is very tall, up to 90cm high, whereas 'Fernleaf', 'Dukat' and 'Superdukat' (more essential oils) are dwarf varieties that grow to around 45cm high, so are perfect for containers. 'Bouquet' is particularly fragrant and is best for seeds.

# How to use

## Dill seed tea

For an after-dinner digestive tea try 1–2 teaspoons of seed, crushed or bruised a little so they absorb water better, in 1 cup of just boiled water and infuse for 10 minutes or so. Add honey to sweeten if you wish.

# ELDERBERRY

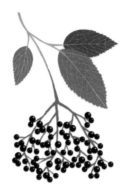

**Other Names** Elderflower, elder.
**Botanical Name** *Sambucus nigra.*
**Family** Adoxaceae (moschatel family).
**Parts Used** Flowers and berries, fresh or dried.
**Plant Properties** Antiviral.
**Uses** To ward off colds and flu, for immune-stimulating properties.
**Preparations** Cordials, soaks or baths, syrups, teas, vinegars of fresh buds.
**Considerations** Any fresh part of this plant taken internally can cause vomiting and nausea, even the fresh flowers (though you'd have to eat a lot of these to feel this effect). The seeds of the berries and leaves are particularly potent; cooking the seed reduces toxicity. Do not eat the leaves.

The elder tree has long been used for medicinal purposes and has a rich folk tradition. The Elder Mother is a spirit who lives in the tree and acts as its guardian. To chop down any elder wood without asking the Elder Mother is to incur her wrath. I remember my mother telling me a half-baked version of the story, which is that you should never make a child's cradle from elder because it will be cursed by the witches. This comes from a Somerset fable of the Elder Mother cursing the wood that had been taken without permission. For years I was terrified of the tree, despite loving the elderflower cordial my mother religiously makes every summer. Denmark, Scotland, Sweden, Sicily and some Slavic countries all believe that elder has magical powers.

Elderflowers are said to help reduce inflammation and increase perspiration. Research shows that they may have anti-inflammatory and antiviral properties. The nectaries are full of sugary secretions for attracting pollinators, but are also known to spread diseases. Essentially, antiviral properties are the flower's way of protecting itself against plant STDs.

When making any elder product, be it elder syrup or elderflower cordial, remove the flowers and the berries from the stems as these are mildly toxic. Use the back of a fork to strip berries from the stem. The flowers are a little trickier: you'll need to lay them out and allow them to dry for several hours so that they can be crumbled from the stem.

The flowers can be taken in tea or cordials or used in salves. It is said that they work particularly well with yarrow and peppermint to shorten the duration and severity of the flu. The unopened flower buds steeped in vinegar are said to be a very effective remedy for sore throats. Pack a jar with the buds, cover with hot cider vinegar and leave to steep. I love using the unripe berries that start to form before the seeds are setting, a couple of weeks after flowering has finished. These steeped in cider vinegar, a little salt and perhaps a touch of sugar – in short, any basic pickling mix – taste just like capers. God only knows if they'll ward off a rasping throat, but they are certainly delicious.

If you eat lots of raw berries and therefore the seeds, then they will make you feel nauseous and eventually you may vomit or have diarrhoea (or both). However, if you gently cook the berries for 3 minutes or so and then carefully press them so they release the juices, you can extract all their goodness. The berries are known for their antiviral properties, and can be used as a mild laxative and a decongestant. They are particularly good at warding off winter flus and colds, and there are many elderberry syrups sold in chemists around the world for this reason. The berries can also be used to make an excellent champagne, which could be considered a tincture of sorts, though I think that any health claim for alcohol is dubious. In any case both elderflower and elderberry champagne are things of beauty.

# How to use

## Elderberry infusions

This tea will make you sweat a lot, so drink plenty of water afterwards. Drink roughly 2 teaspoons of dried flowers or 2–3 heads of fresh flowers in hot water up to three times a day.

Traditionally before drinking you should sit in a bath with elderberry flowers in a muslin bag. Soak for 20 minutes, drink the tea and then go to bed wrapped in an extra blanket and apparently you'll sweat out your sins (or that cold). Replace liquids by drinking plenty of water.

## Elderberry syrup

Cook the fresh or dried berries with a little water until soft, then press through a jelly bag. Measure the juice and add equal parts honey, then bring back to the boil, remove from the heat and store in an airtight rubber-sealed preserving jar or similar in the fridge. Take 1–2 teaspoons four times a day throughout the winter. This should store for 4–6 weeks in the fridge or you can freeze the mixture in ice cubes. Add ginger, cinnamon and thyme to the syrup for flavour if you wish.

# EUCALYPTUS

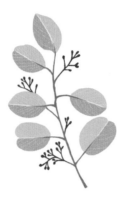

**Other Name** Gum tree.
**Botanical Name** *Eucalyptus* species.
**Family** Myrtaceae (myrtle family).
**Parts Used** Leaves, gum.
**Plant Properties** Antimicrobial, decongestant, antiviral.
**Uses** Clearing sinuses, expectorant for respiratory congestion, antiseptic, antibacterial.

**Preparations** Steam inhalations, strewing herb for baths.
**Considerations** The essential oil is powerful stuff and should never be used undiluted as it contains cineole, a skin irritant. A steam inhalation of leaves is safe for adults.

**Should not be used during pregnancy or by children under four.**

While eucalyptus may not strictly be a herb, I am including it here not because I expect you to grow it, but because it's so easy, particularly in towns, to find a tree to forage from. Most parks have a eucalyptus or two with plenty of leaves low enough to pick. All eucalyptus are evergreen and have two types of leaves:

juvenile and adult. The adult leaves possess greater amounts of essential oils.

The *Eucalyptus* genus is large: around 515 different species. The most common ornamental plants are the Tasmanian blue gum, *E. globulus*, which tends to be found in southern, milder locations in the UK and is commercially grown for its essential oils, and the cider gum, *E. gunnii*. The adult leaves of the cider gum are blue-green, long and slender and hang downwards from a single stalk. The juvenile leaves are blue, round and unstalked. The flower buds are cone-shaped and grouped together in sets of three on short stakes. The flowers are full of fluffy white or red stamens that are hugely attractive to bees and are honey-scented.

The essential oil is widely available from pharmacies and health food shops. It should be diluted with a neutral base, such as olive oil or jojoba oil, then it can be used on cuts and wounds for its anti-microbial properties or as an insect repellent.

# How to forage

The leaves and young twigs can be used fresh or dried and are best harvested in spring or summer.

# How to use

Adult leaves can be added to a bowl of hot water to create a steam inhalation. Depending on the size of the leaves, usually three or four are fine. I often add a handful of leaves to a bath, particularly if I'm also adding salt. This makes an antiseptic bath that can help relieve congestion, clear sinuses and aid breathing. It smells divine and I personally find it both restores and enlivens. Before bed I add lavender flowers to my bath; if I need to wake myself up to go out dancing, I add eucalyptus. You can also hang small branches of eucalyptus under your showerhead for a similar effect.

# FENNEL

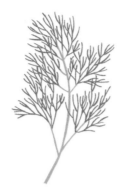

**Botanical Name** *Foeniculum vulgare.*

**Family** Apiaceae (carrot family).

**Parts Used** Leaves, flowers and seeds, fresh or dried.

**Plant Properties** Antimicrobial, antispasmodic, antiflammatory, aromatic, carminative, diuretic, stimulates menstrual flow, stomach-soothing.

**Uses** Indigestion, can relieve diarrhoea and safe to use in young children, relieves bloating and gas, is said to sweeten and increase breast milk, freshens breath.

**Preparations** Culinary, infusions, teas.

**Considerations** Fennel seed is a natural emmenagogue, meaning it helps stimulate or increase menstrual flow. Do not confuse it with the giant fennel, *Ferula communis*, which is found in the Mediterranean and is very poisonous. You'll notice that grazing goats and sheep will avoid it like the plague for this reason.

**Not to be used in pregnancy.**

Fennel is loved around the world for both its culinary and medicinal properties. Indigenous to the shores of the Mediterranean, it is also found worldwide, often naturalized in dry soils near the coast, riverbeds or motorways. The banks of many of Britain's busiest roads are often lined with fennel, good for brave bees and hoverflies, but not much use to the forager due to all that pollution.

Fennel's seeds and leaves both have a strong, clean flavour of aniseed, coming from the aromatic compound anethole. Fennel seed is used in the production of akvavit and absinthe. The seed is a rich source of protein, dietary fibre and minerals, including calcium, iron and manganese. Seeds can simply be chewed after a meal to sweeten the breath. They can also be toasted to impart a nutty flavour that works well in tomato-based sauces or scattered over roasted vegetables.

Chiefly fennel is used to decrease bloating and gas. It can be used on infants with colic; a weak tea fed by the teaspoon is widely documented. If breastfeeding, then the mother can take the tea, which will stimulate milk production and improve the digestibility of the milk. It can also be used to treat menstrual cramps.

Fennel has long been used for eye health and a compress made from the tea can be used to help with conjunctivitis and inflammation of the eyelid.

The tea is a great after-dinner drink and can be combined with other digestive herbs, such as caraway or coriander (see tea for digestion recipe on page 84).

## How to grow

The herb fennel, as opposed to the bulb fennel that you slice for salads, is a perennial and will grow in a wide range of soils as long as they are not too wet over winter. If you have heavy clay, then add grit to your planting hole to improve drainage. They do best in full sun and will grow in thin urban soils very happily. They will self-seed, though they dislike being moved once established. A bronze form, *Foeniculum vulgare* 'Purpureum', is highly ornamental and the seed can be used just the same way as the straight species.

Herb fennel can be started from seed. It does need to be fresh as seed that has been stored for more than a year tends to lose viability. Sow in spring, under heat, either on a sunny windowsill or in a propagator, and prick out when large enough to handle. Young plants are often very cheap and widely available both via mail order or at garden centres. As they are extremely drought-tolerant they are a good plant for a sunny balcony or courtyard. They grow very successfully in pots, as long as they can get their roots down, so choose a pot with a minimum of 30cm diameter and depth. Fennel is hardy, dying back in autumn and appearing again in mid-spring. Slugs can devour young plants, particularly if they sit in shade. If slugs are a problem for you, pot on young plants until you have a decent specimen, then plant it out.

# How to use

## Fennel tea

For culinary purposes young green seeds are powerful, but for tea, tisanes and infusions, dried seeds are perfect. Crushing the seeds before use will release their oil.

For a weak tea that can be drunk up to three times a day use 1 tablespoon/6g of seeds in 90ml of water. Cover the seeds with just boiled water and let the mixture steep for 5 minutes. Strain and add honey if desired.

For a sore throat or the start of a cold add lemon balm to this mixture to increase its anti-inflammatory properties. Adults can drink this tea up to three times a day, but infants and young children will need only 1 teaspoon (5ml). For colic treatment it's best to consult a clinical herbalist for specialized dosing.

# FEVERFEW

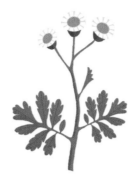

**Other Name** Bachelor's button.

**Botanical Name** *Tanacetum parthenium.*

**Family** Asteraceae (sunflower or daisy family).

**Parts Used** Leaves and flowers, fresh or dried.

**Plant Properties** Analgesic, anti-inflammatory, nervine.

**Uses** Migraines.

**Preparations** Direct consumption, teas.

**Considerations** Can cause mouth sores and ulcerations if regularly used in strong doses. It may interfere with aspirin and other anticoagulant medications.

**Not to be used in pregnancy.**

Feverfew is a very pretty white and yellow daisy with a nice frilly leaf. It's a carefree sort and once in your garden pops up all over the place. The leaves, when crushed, have a strong aromatic, slightly bitter scent that is very much present when you eat them, and this flavour will linger on your tongue. You do get used to the taste after a while, but add leaves sparingly to salads or bread and butter sandwiches. They add little flavour other than bitterness, but it's a simple and effective way to take this herb.

Feverfew gets its name because it is said to reduce a fever and it is well known as a folk remedy for migraines. The jury is a little out on whether this works – it did go through a stage of being denigrated by orthodox medicine – but new evidence shows that its long-held reputation is backed by scientific evidence. It seems that for most people feverfew doesn't work if you take it when a headache or migraine is present, but there's some evidence to show that taking a very low dose on a daily basis might be beneficial in preventing headaches. It is said to work because of its anti-inflammatory effect as well as its strong bitter digestives (that's those leaves in a salad), which help with the nausea and vomiting often associated with migraines.

## How to grow

Sow in spring, either direct or in seed trays, in full sun. This one loves to grow from the thinnest of cracks and in path edges. The seed is tiny and needs to be sown on soil or compost surface. Prick out when large enough to handle. Let it choose its position in your garden or pots and cut back immediately after flowering if you don't want it to spread. You can find a very pretty double form of feverfew, *Tanacetum parthenium* 'Flore Pleno', as well as one with a variegated yellow and green leaf, *T. parthenium* 'Aureum', and there's a very strange but beguiling variety, *T. parthenium* 'Malmesbury', which has stubby petals and a yellow centre to the flower, that looks like a cartoon drawing of a friendly sun.

# How to use

For long-term relief of headaches you should eat 3 leaves a day. This can be done all at once in a bread and butter sandwich or you can eat them over the course of the day. They are so bitter that you might choose the latter. Some people are very sensitive to the Asteraceae family and feverfew has been known to cause mouth blisters if eaten directly. The idea is that the bread and butter tempers this issue.

# GARLIC

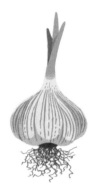

**Botanical Name** *Allium sativum.*

**Family** Amaryllidaceae (lily family).

**Parts Used** Bulb, cloves, scapes (unopened flowers).

**Plant Properties** Stimulating, antimicrobial, carminative, vermifugal, expectorant.

**Uses** Fungal infections, bacterial infections, digestion, parasites, cold and flu remedy.

**Preparations** Culinary.

**Considerations** Some laboratory studies suggest too much garlic can thin the blood and therefore if you are on warfarin or other blood-thinning medicine, then you should consult your doctor about your consumption. If you were to eat one to two entire bulbs of garlic daily for a long period of time, then you would see some harmful effects, such as anaemia and bowel flora disruption. I can't even start to imagine how someone could regularly eat that much garlic, but you never know . . .

Les Blanks suggested that when theatres screened his legendary documentary *Garlic Is as Good as Ten Mothers*, they should roast several heads of garlic slowly in a toaster oven so that approximately halfway through the film, unbeknownst to the audience, the theatre would start to reek of cooking garlic. A brilliant idea, but when I tried this at a local film festival I just smoked the audience out. Still, they came back, because it's a truly wonderful film. The title refers to a Spanish saying that 'Garlic is as good as ten mothers . . . for keeping the girls away'. And anyone who's consumed a lot of it will know that it makes not only your breath, but your skin too, reek of the stinking rose. It's this all-pervasive quality that makes it a potentially powerful medicine.

Many think of garlic as being a Mediterranean plant, particularly Italian, but its true origins are probably somewhere in central and south-western Asia. Plenty have sought to discover the original home of the first garlic plant, but it's been grown around the globe since antiquity, appearing in nearly every cuisine in the world, so pinning down the original source may be impossible. There are two subspecies of *Allium sativum*, and ten major groups of varieties and hundreds of cultivars. It's not possible to say whether one of these is better than the other for health, but without doubt those that are grown organically are better for the planet.

As long as garlic has been eaten it has also been used for medicine. From the bubonic plague and dropsy to smallpox and gangrene during the First and Second World Wars, garlic has been used to cure a whole host of medical complaints. Galen of Pergamon, a physician, surgeon and philosopher considered to be one of the most accomplished of medical researchers in antiquity, considered it a *theriaca rusticorum*, a 'rustic's theriac; a cure all for ills'. A theriac being a sort of treacly medicinal concoction that was used for poisonous bites.

Modern-day science can't decide how it feels about garlic. Meta-study after meta-study conclude that evidence is contradictory: it does, it doesn't. And then there are confounding factors such as limitation in interpretation. The jury is out on whether it definitively helps with cardiovascular diseases, some cancers and common colds. Still, garlic tastes delicious and nearly every herbal text extols its antimicrobial properties, and this much is validated by science. Garlic may not be a 'cure all' for major diseases, but it will help maintain a healthy gut flora. It can reduce bad bacteria and fungi, such as the yeast candida, *Candida albicans*, and streptococcus, and it, along with many other foods that make up a healthy diet, will stimulate your immune system. Interestingly, however, Buddhist temples do not use garlic in their food (along with other pungent food in the same family: leeks, chives, green onions, bulb onions) because it may overstimulate the liver and not aid with concentration for meditation.

Garlic contains allicin, which when chopped or crushed gives garlic its pungent smell. Allicin is antibacterial, antifungal and antiparasitic and so is produced as part of a defence mechanism against attacks by pest and diseases on the garlic plant. Allicin is broken down by our bodies into compounds that pass into the bloodstream via the intestines. Once in the bloodstream the only way to get rid of allicin is to sweat it out or pass it through your lungs, hence why your breath and skin smell after eating quantities of garlic.

Garlic naturally thins the blood and it's also antispasmodic and hypotensive, so will lower blood pressure, another contributor to heart disease. Garlic also contains inulin, a starch used to store energy in the bulb. Plants that use and store inulin don't tend to store other forms of starch, such as carbohydrates. Some people are very sensitive to garlic and the rest of the allium family, and one of the effects of this may be due to the inulin, which can cause diarrhoea, cramping, bloating and intestinal discomfort. For the rest of us inulin is a very good prebiotic. Prebiotics are compounds in food that induce the growth of beneficial microorganisms, such as bacteria and fungi in the gut. Inulin resists absorption in the upper gastrointestinal tract, only breaking down in the large intestine, where it nourishes the gut microflora. In short, it's great for gut health and most traditional diets include garlic for this reason. For garlic's therapeutic properties to be fully exploited it must be eaten raw; heating destroys much of its goodness.

# How to grow

Garlic is so wonderfully easy to grow. Stick a single clove, pointed end up, in the ground or a pot in autumn and watch it grow through the cold, wet months to ripen in midsummer. A single clove produces a bulb of four to ten new cloves. Garlic plants need to go through a cold period for bulb initiation to occur. If it spends fewer than ten nights under 10°C/50°F, the cloves won't form properly and the plant will produce a single large bulb that won't store. In the northern hemisphere there are two periods of planting garlic: in autumn and in spring. In the autumn the last of the lingering warmth starts growth off before winter appears. I usually plant between the last two weeks of October and the first two of November. You can plant again in February, though you do need to make sure you are planting a variety that is suitable for this period. Varieties are marked for either autumn planting, spring planting or both.

If you have heavy soil, particularly clay, plant in a ridge of soil that will draw water away from the bulb so it doesn't rot over winter. Garlic is a hungry, competitive plant that does best when widely spaced. Allow your planted clove a diameter of 18–25cm to itself to ensure decent-sized cloves and feed from late April through to early June, either by top-dressing with a mulch, such as home-made compost in mid-spring, or with liquid feed, such as seaweed, comfrey or nettle tea. When the tops start to yellow and bend, the garlic is ready to be pulled. Don't make the mistake of yanking it up without gently teasing it with a fork beforehand, otherwise you'll just be left holding the yellowing stems and will have to root around in the soil for the bulk. Also, the neck is very sensitive until it's been dried and damaging it can help rot to set in.

Dry your garlic somewhere warm and airy, such as a polytunnel, greenhouse, garage, barn or shed. Avoid drying in your kitchen: the smell will be too pungent. Once the bulbs are completely dry you can process them for storage. Only soft-neck types will plait; hard-neck garlic, where there's a hard flower spike in the centre of the bulb, are not suitable for a traditional garlic plait, and need to have the stem cut back to just above the bulb, roots trimmed and be stored somewhere cool and dry. I like to keep mine in a wicker basket.

Storage of garlic depends very much on the cultivar, and early-maturing ones don't tend to store as long as later-maturing cultivars. A general rule of thumb is that soft-neck varieties tend to store a little longer than hard-neck ones. If you get into growing garlic in a big way, it makes a lot of sense to grow a range of cultivars to best exploit flavour, heat and storage.

If you suffer from leek moth or allium leaf miner, both pests that mine into the skin between the clove and bulb and pupate there, then you will need to cover your garlic from the start of planting till harvest with a fine-mesh netting to stop the pesky females from laying their eggs. Make sure the mesh netting is buried round the edges so there are no gaps.

# How to use

The simplest way to use garlic is just to eat it. I probably eat up to four cloves most days, which says a lot about my cooking, I guess. How you work with garlic will affect the allicin; minced garlic is much stronger in flavour than a whole clove gently roasted. The finer you chop, the more heat will come through. Raw garlic is pungent and thirst-inducing and can make you feel sick if you eat it alone; cooked garlic is trans-formed and easier to consume. For its purest medicinal properties you do need to eat it raw. If you are trying to ward off a cold with garlic, then consuming it throughout the day rather than in one go makes more sense. The simplest way to eat raw garlic for such reasons is to rub it on toast and smother it in olive oil, a delicious medicinal snack. If you can't stomach raw fresh garlic, then fermenting it in honey or making it into an oxymel is a far more palatable option.

## Garlic honey

Peel 15–20 cloves of garlic. Cover with 120ml of honey, ensuring all cloves are covered by 0.5cm or so. Let sit for 24 hours before using. You'll notice the honey gets much runnier as it draws out the moisture from the cloves. After a while the garlic will become chewy and tough as all the water is drawn out and the whole mixture will start to ferment. Don't worry about this; it's just adding to the flavour profile. The mixture will store forever: I have year-old batches. However, if you don't like the flavour of fermented honey, make small batches and keep it in the fridge (which slows down fermentation).

You can chew whole cloves of garlic to ward off a cold if you are brave, but it might be more pleasant to take a teaspoon of the honey infusion when you feel a winter cold coming along. I also use this honey when making an oxymel (see page 115) or a honey and Dijon mustard salad dressing.

I also use garlic honey for athlete's foot. I've no scientific evidence for this at all, other than garlic is a powerful anti-fungicide and honey is great for sore skin, particularly pressure sores. I rub the honey mixture on before bed and wash it off the following morning.

## Fermented garlic

I love using garlic along with chillies to flavour brine for fermentation. Cucumbers, carrots, kimchi, vegetables, everything from Brussels sprouts to whole chillies get at least two whole cloves of garlic in the brine mix. Eating the cloves left at the end of the pickle jar is one of my favourite treats. I'd fight anyone for those.

## Fire cider

Fire cider is as old as the hills, though the first written version is credited to herbalist Rosemary Gladstar. This is reason alone to consult her work; her books are wonderful – read them all! The recommended dosage for preventing a cold is to take 1 tablespoon three times a day when you feel the start of a cold coming on. If you've got a cold, then take this every couple of hours. Fire cider also makes an excellent vinegar for salad dressings and works very well as a marinade for meat and tofu.

100g minced onion

100g grated horseradish (wear swimming goggles and do this outside, if possible, as fresh horseradish straight from the ground contains lots of mustard oils)

100g minced garlic (around 15 cloves)

25g ginger

25g peeled and diced turmeric

1 small chilli, split in half, or ½ teaspoon dried chilli pepper

2 tablespoons thyme, chopped

2 tablespoons rosemary, chopped

2 teaspoons whole black peppercorns

½ lemon, sliced into rounds

285g raw honey

630ml raw cider vinegar

Place all the dry ingredients and vegetables in a 1-litre rubber-sealed preserving jar and cover with the honey. Then fill the jar with the vinegar. Ensure there's enough vinegar to keep everything submerged and stir well to get rid of any air bubbles. Cover the jar with a glass lid. If you have a metal one, then use parchment paper between the jar mouth and the lid to prevent the metal corroding with the vinegar. Let the jar sit for 2–3 weeks, shaking it occasionally to mix. Strain the vinegar into a clear airtight jar and use up within the year.

## Oxymel

An oxymel is an ancient recipe, originally a sweet vinegar or wine, the name coming from the Greek *oxy*, meaning an acid, and *mel*, honey. Oxymels were big in the late Renaissance pharmacopoeias (official lists of medicinal drugs, their effectiveness and uses), and persisted into Victorian times as a widely used medical prescription. Often oxymels were used to make tart or bitter herbs more palatable; you can stick almost anything you care into an oxymel. Drink a teaspoon a day or use it as a delicious salad dressing, or add it to hot water or top it up with sparkling water for a refreshing drink with floral summer herbs such as basil, mint or hyssop. To make any sort of health claims for an oxymel is pretty ludicrous other than the obvious: these are all good ingredients and food is medicine.

Fresh thyme, sage, rosemary, hyssop, basil, lemon basil, holy basil or lemon balm (if using dried herbs, use in lower quantities)

Cinnamon
Garlic cloves
Local, unpasteurized honey
Raw cider vinegar, preferably with the mother

Oxymels are generally made with one part vinegar to two parts herbs and two parts honey. However, feel free to adjust to taste. Fill a quarter of a jar with herbs, garlic and cinnamon and then top it up with parts honey and vinegar. Cover the jar with a non-metallic lid; the vinegar will corrode the lid otherwise. If you have a metallic lid, use parchment paper between the metal and the liquid. Shake the mixture once a day for two weeks. Strain out the mash and then store in the fridge. The oxymel will last for a year.

# HAWTHORN

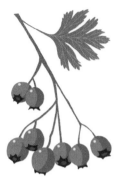

**Other Names** Haw, May tree, hawberry, bread and cheese tree.

**Botanical Names** *Crataegus monogyna* (American), *Crataegus laevigata* (English or Midland hawthorn).

**Family** Rosaceae (rose family).

**Parts Used** Leaves, flowers, fruit.

**Plant Properties** Antispasmodic, diuretic, tonic, astringent, sedative, vasodilatory (opens the blood vessels).

**Uses** Improves the heart and cardiovascular system, for the treatment of diarrhoea, and relieves anxiety.

**Preparations** Culinary, infusions, teas.

**Considerations** Should not be taken with other heart medicines without consulting a medical practitioner.

Hawthorn is said to be food for the heart and it is widely used by herbalists to treat the heart and circulatory system. Most of us won't have a hawthorn tree of our own to harvest from, but every hedgerow, park, wayside or verge will do so. Hawthorn, or May blossom, are ubiquitous trees at the edges of our world. They can be scrappy, hidden in a clipped hedge or marvellously weather-beaten, growing craggy and windswept with the weather.

Hawthorns are a large group and there are many species and even more hybrids. On the whole hybrids are good to eat but considered less medicinally effective. Some species have berries so large that they look like crab apples. Travelling through Kazakhstan in autumn, we saw endless roadside stalls selling the crab apple-sized berries of *Crataegus pontica*, the ponti hawthorn, which were bright yellow and orange, and perfect snacks for travelling, tasting somewhat like apples with a hint of papaya.

Hawthorn flowers and leaves are known to be rich in plant pigments called flavonoids and, along with the berries, have gained recognition as being a potent heart remedy that improves coronary circulation by dilating the blood vessels. Preparations of leaves and flowers of certain species of *Crataegus* have been used in remedies for cardiac disease and strengthening the aging heart since the first century CE. Today Crataegus extract is a recognized treatment for heart failure and has undergone numerous clinical trials proving its efficacy as an add-on therapy. However, the doses and preparation for such things is way beyond the kitchen dabbler.

The berries are also said to be very effective against diarrhoea due to their astringent properties. Hawthorn blossom and leaves steeped as a tea have long been used to calm a fluttering heart. The blossom tea is certainly pretty to watch swirling around a glass teapot, and that in itself is calming.

Hawthorns often have sharp, straight thorns on their branches and the trees can grow up to 9 metres. The leaves are deciduous and lobed with serrated margins. The flowers are fragrant and often white or pink, forming in clusters.

# How to grow

Hawthorn is readily and easily available to forage. However, if you're looking for a small tree for the bottom of your garden, it's a fine one to consider with its lovely flowers, berries and autumn colour. The American haw, *C. monogyna*, with its large red berries is very attractive.

# How to use

## Hawthorn tea

An infusion of leaves and flowers can be drunk up to three times a day and is a good calming tea. Use 1–2 teaspoons per cup and steep for 12–15 minutes, covered. It can be mixed with other herbs, such as oat straw or lime blossom, to give it a little more flavour.

## For culinary use

Hawthorn berries make an excellent jam or sauce that you might use the same way you would a ketchup or brown sauce. Either will preserve some of those 'good heart' properties. If you find a large American, Mediterranean or Asian species of hawthorn growing in your park and are confident in your identification, the haw makes an excellent snack; simply chew the berries and spit out the seeds.

You can eat young hawthorn leaves and their buds, which taste of a hint of 'pepper and salt', and their folk name of the bread and cheese plant reflects that they work well in a bread and butter sandwich, as long as you don't expect the cheese part! The flowers are also edible and work well with sweet things and fruit salads. The flowers are said to bring fairies into the house.

## For medicinal use

Traditionally a poultice of pulped leaves or fruit was used to draw out thorns and splinters and heal whitlows. The astringent nature of the fruit and leaves certainly make this a logical benefit.

# HOPS

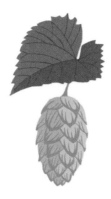

**Other Name** Common hops.

**Botanical Name** *Humulus lupulus.*

**Family** Cannabaceae (hemp family).

**Parts Used** Strobili, the bright green cone-like flowers.

**Plant Properties** Nervine, sedative, tonic, astringent.

**Uses** Calms and relaxes nerves and organs, strong sedative.

**Preparations** Herb pillows, poultices, teas.

**Considerations** Hops contain phytoestrogen, the plant equivalent of oestrogen, and there's some evidence to suggest that long-term use in women might cause irregular menstruation and increase oestrogen in the body, which in turn is linked with breast cancer. There's also anecdotal evidence that this phytoestrogen may reduce male sex drive and cause 'beer breasts'.

As hops have a gentle sedative effect they can be used to treat mild anxiety, but if you suffer from depression, speak to your doctor or registered herbalist first as there is evidence to show that hops might be counterproductive and even exacerbate depression.

The long and short of this is that hops cones are not recommended for long-term daily use. If you find the plant particularly helpful for a good night's sleep, a hops pillow might be a more gentle long-term alternative.

Hops cones are dangerous to both cats and dogs if consumed, so make sure any spent hops and hops pillows are kept out of paws' reach.

---

**Hops tea is not suitable for pregnant or breastfeeding mothers and should not be used on children under two years old.**

---

Hops are one of the key ingredients for beer and bedtime, perhaps in that order. Beer actually uses a surprisingly small amount of hops; they simply flavour the mash used to brew beer. Strobili, hops' cone-like flowers, have to be picked at peak ripeness. As soon as they turn a bright lime-green and are covered in a sticky yellow dust-like substance known as lupulin then they are ready to pick. Try to pick them before the cones start to brown at the edges. Once dried and put in an airtight container hops will store for about 6 months, after which they will lose their potency. This container must be kept cool and away from temperature fluctuations.

The smell of hops is strong and seductive. I collected numerous seed heads in Kazakhstan and started the process of harvesting the seed in the long car journeys through the dusty brown steppe landscape between mountains. The steppe is a low, gently undulating landscape that looks almost desert-like in autumn, repetitious apart from the golden eagles hanging out by the endless straight motorways waiting for roadkill. Even past their peak the aroma was so strong we all started to drift off, my fingers sticky from collecting the seed. My brown paper bags of scales and dried leaves had to be banished to the boot in several layers of plastic bags so that we could all keep our eyes open.

The flavour and aroma of hops is rated by its 'alpha', the percentage of total alpha acids, the compounds essential for making beer taste as it does, compared to the dry weight. The stronger the alpha, the more pronounced the bitter flavour. Likewise, the higher the alpha percentage, the stronger the medicine. However, truly bitter hops are quite hard to drink. It's possible to make a tea of just hops, but it's not pleasant, so for that reason most people like to add other herbs to make them more palatable or use them in a pillow to drift off to the delicious odour.

## How to grow

Hops are perennial climbers; in the wild they grow up to 6 metres and have a large root mass. Although there are dwarf varieties, hops are not really suitable for small spaces. For beer making you need to treat your hops like queens and give them a deep, long, fertile root run on a south or south-west aspect with support for the vines to grow up. Usually only 2–4 shoots are chosen to grow up the string or support, so that there is enough energy to create large hops. As hops are dioecious, meaning that male and female flowers are grown on separate plants, you'll need female plants for tea. A reputable seller will send you virus- and disease-free female stock. Your plant won't produce many flowers in its first year as it concentrates on making a good root run. Many hops plants are sold bare root in the autumn; when planting these dig a hole large enough for the long roots and make sure you cover the crown of the plant with mulch to protect it from frost in its first year.

You can also grow hops from seed, which is my preference. This method takes an extra year or so to grow sturdy plants. Hops seed will need cold scarification, a simulation of a winter under snow to encourage germination. The easiest way to do this is to put the seed in an equal amount of moist sand or between sheets of damp kitchen towel and refrigerate for four to eight weeks in a clear plastic bag (a freezer one is ideal), labelling and dating the bag. After the chilling period, sow the seeds in good-quality peat-free compost at around 20°C/68°F, either on a warm windowsill or in a heat propagator. Germination should take two to four weeks; prick out when seedlings are large enough to handle. If you start the germination process off in January, your plants should be large enough to go outside as the season warms up.

Hops should be picked when they are green and slightly sticky. The stems of hops plants are pretty vicious scratchy things that will mark your arms, so wear long sleeves and gloves to protect your skin. Pick early in the day before cones start releasing the dust-like lupulin. The female cones are often hidden under the leaves, so be prepared to really get in there. You can hack down whole shoots to collect the hops as it's very hard to kill this rambunctious plant. I have three hops plants: one that is taking over my shed roof and two that grow up and over a pergola into a tree. Three are far too many plants for one person's tea needs. There is a variety called 'Prima Donna' that only grows to 2.4 metres and is perfect for growing along fences.

# How to use

## Hops tea for bedtime

Make a basic tea or infusion by combining 2 teaspoons of dried hops in 1 cup of water. Allow to steep for 4 minutes, then strain and drink. It's quite a bitter concoction, so add honey if necessary. You can add all sorts of other flavours to hops tea: lemongrass, ginger, camomile, lavender and oat straw all work well, either in combinations or alone.

1 part camomile flowers

2 parts lemon balm

2 parts lemongrass (fresh if possible)

2 parts ginger (fresh)

½ part lavender flowers

¼ part hops flowers

250ml water

Parts are measured by volume, not weight.

Drink 1 cup before bed. This tea will store for 6 months in an airtight container.

## For culinary use

If you grow your own, you can also sample the deliciousness that is hops shoots in early spring. The first few shoots, when they are pencil length, can be cut, as the plant will reshoot again. These can be briefly steamed or sautéed in butter or oil and are delicious with a sprinkling of salt. They taste fresh and green with a good bite, a hint of asparagus and something a little nutty. They are used in risottos or with fettuccine mixed with other spring greens, such as dandelions

and wild chicory, or mixed into an omelette or frittata they are a surprisingly versatile spring green.

## Hops pillow

You can make a small hops pillow by combining hops cones with
lavender and/or camomile flowers. The simplest way to do this is to
make a small 10 by 10cm case that you place inside an ordinary
pillowcase.

# HORSERADISH

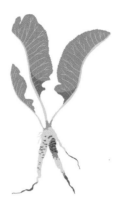

**Botanical Name** *Amoracia rusticana.*
**Family** Brassicaceae.
**Parts Used** Leaves, flowers, roots.
**Plant Properties** Stimulant, antimicrobial, antibacterial, diuretic, stimulant.

**Uses** For colds, and clears sinuses and chest infections.
**Preparations** Condiments, poultices.
**Considerations** Avoid eating if horseradish upsets your stomach or causes gastrointestinal discomfort, or if you have stomach or intestinal ulcers.

When I was a child my mother used to send me off to a lush bank down a country lane near our house where horseradish grew in abundance. I'd dig up the first 5 cm or so of root, also known as a thong, with a stick, twisting it off so we could have horseradish sauce with our Sunday beef. The same bank also grew mint, so sometimes I'd collect that for the sauce for roast lamb. That bank is forever forged with Sunday lunch in my memory. Anyway, the horseradish grew in fertile, damp ground next to a spring (which is why the mint liked it too), a perfect spot for fat roots. Horseradish grown on poor, thin or stony soil is often tough, stringy and a pain to prepare.

Horseradish is a fiery fiend. If you're going to grate the stuff, be prepared to don swimming goggles and go outside to do the job, otherwise you'll feel like you've mustard-gassed your kitchen! It's a powerful herb that needs to be used with caution because it has such a strong afterburn. Still, I, for one, love the flavour and it's an effective food preservative; the freshly grated root is incredibly antimicrobial and protects against bacterial pathogens.

Horseradish has a long herbal history, appearing in Greek, Roman and Renaissance herbals, though today its medicinal uses have largely been forgotten. The name comes not from the animal, but from an archaic use of 'horse', meaning strong or coarse, and it was thought to be in the same genus as radish. Thus the name recalls its giant roots.

Horseradish contains a number of volatile oils, including the mustard oil, allyl isothiocyanate, which gives it its distinctive pungent smell. It is high in vitamin C when used fresh. Eating it clears the sinuses and helps treat the common cold, but it has also traditionally been used as a remedy for rheumatism.

## How to grow

Think wisely before you plant a horseradish as it's very hard to get rid of once settled into its home. I planted a tiny root thong years ago on my allotment, only to decide it was the wrong place, and ten years later I am still digging it out! This can be avoided by growing the root in an old plastic bin or similar with holes punched into the bottom, and plunge this into the ground. This will not only keep those power-ful roots contained, but you can fill it with compost and ensure lovely long, straight roots. Like carrots, horseradish grown on stony ground produces twisted roots that are a bother to clean and peel.

# How to use

## For culinary use

Horseradish is delicious when prepared with either vinegar or cream and used as a condiment. Grated and mixed with cider vinegar, so that the horseradish is completely covered, and with a good pinch of salt, it can be stored in the fridge for up to 3 months. Add cream to this mix to make a traditional horseradish sauce or mix it in with mustard for a fiery condiment. The raw horseradish will stimulate the digestive system and protects against food pathogens, which is perhaps one of the reasons it is such a common traditional ingredient in central and eastern European dishes. It is a key ingredient in fire cider (see page 114) and is taken in the winter to ward off colds and flu.

The young leaves, when still soft and tender and no more than 20cm long, are delicious, with a gentle heat and only a touch of bite. These can be added to vinegar or used in salads.

The flowers are spicy and pungent and make an interesting add-ition to salad.

## Horseradish poultice

The root will burn skin and can cause blistering, so put down a thick layer of salve or ointment first and then wrap the root in layers of cotton. Remove the poultice the minute you feel the skin start to burn. Horseradish should never be used on children for this reason. It's more of a curiosity than a recommendation because of its potential to burn.

# HYSSOP

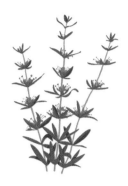

**Botanical Name** *Hyssopus officinalis.*
**Family** Lamiaceae (mint family).
**Parts Used** Leaves and flowers without stems.

**Plant Properties** Stimulant, expectorant, antiviral, diuretic, anti-inflammatory, diaphoretic.
**Uses** Coughs, colds.
**Preparations** Infusions, syrups, teas.

---

### Hyssop should be avoided during pregnancy.

---

Hyssop is such a wonderfully old-fashioned-sounding name, and it's a bit of an old-fashioned herb that you don't hear nearly enough about these days, which is silly. It's easy to grow and wonderful to use. Its history goes back to classical antiquity. Hyssop hails from the Mediterranean and is a small evergreen, willow-leaved shrub. It has a pleasant, slightly medicinal perfume that, if smelt in the midday sun, has a hit of turpentine. The leaves have a long history of use in cooking; the flavour has strong notes of mint followed by floral traces and coal tar and a lingering taste of grass when fresh.

Hyssop is one of the main ingredients of zaatar, along with sumac. It also makes up one of the ingredients of the liqueur Chartreuse. It produces a rich and aromatic honey and attracts all manner of pollinators. Although it may not seem the most obvious choice for a herb garden, I believe that hyssop is one of those plants that every garden should have, for once you start to use it in cooking and herbal medicine you quickly come to love its reliable nature. This is, in part, because hyssop is as tough as old boots; so long as it has a sunny position with its feet in free-draining soil it will come through rain, wind and winter snows to be crowned in lovely blue, pink and, more rarely, white fragrant flowers come summer. It's these flowers that you use for tea and medicine.

## How to grow

Hyssop is easy enough to grow as long as it has a south- or west-facing spot and is in fertile, well-drained soil. It does very well on chalk and loam, but if you have neither add up to 50 per cent grit to the planting hole. With time (around five to ten years) it will grow up to 1 metre tall and a similar size in spread. When you buy a small 9cm plant it is easy to be tricked into thinking that it will stay neat and plant it near the edge of a border. Instead, think of it like a large lavender plant and give it space to grow to stature. Regularly harvesting will keep it in shape. However, if you are finding it grows a little too unruly, prune it back by a third, making sure to remove shoots that have flowered. It also grows very successfully in a large pot of at least 30cm diameter.

You can harvest hyssop twice a year: once in mid-spring, when you might be pruning it anyway (see above), and again just as it comes into peak flower. The latter is preferable because you'll get both leaf and flower. Harvest carefully for all parts bruise easily and discolour. The best method is to cut whole stems down by a third and hang your bunches somewhere cool, airy and, most importantly, out of direct sunlight. Make sure the bundles are not too tightly tied as airflow is required to conserve the gentle aroma. Once dried remove the leaves and flowers from the stem and store in an airtight container.

Anise hyssop, *Agastache foeniculum*, is a perennial herb from North America that has remarkably similar blue flowers. However, the leaves look similar to mint, and have a distinct, sharp anise scent and white undersides. The plant was traditionally used by First Nation people to treat coughs and colds in much the same way hyssop is used. It has similar requirements, needing full sun and well-drained soil. It is faster-growing so may develop mildew if planted in too tightly or with poor air circulation. Never use mildewed leaves for tea. In the UK it is somewhat tender and may need to be treated as an annual. It's very attractive and well worth growing, but as hyssop is hardier and more long-lived, it's perhaps more useful if you are limited for space.

*Agastache rugosa*, known as liquorice mint or Korean mint, or purple giant hyssop, is widely grown in East Asia, where it is used in both cooking and Chinese traditional medicine. It tastes sweet with gentle notes of liquorice and a hint of mint and basil. It is used in Korean cuisine, often added at the last minute to dishes, and is a key ingredient in Korean pancakes. Its leaves also make a very calming drink, which is used in Chinese medicine to relieve nausea, vomiting, poor appetite and headaches, and to treat morning sickness. It's a good tea for a hangover. As a tea it is somewhat spicy, ending in notes of liquorice and aniseed, though I can't say the smell is that wonderful.

Korean mint grows best with sun; the flavour is somewhat dampened by too much shade. Once established it's quite tough, but it does need damp feet to get there and will not do well in thin, parched soils. It's easy to grow from seed sown in spring in a heated propagator. It flowers from July to September and is a perennial, but it is not hardy and will usually die at temperatures of around −5°C/23°F. In warmer, better protected areas it will make it through the winter, particularly if mulched well in autumn. Cut back after flowering. It is also possible to take cuttings in spring, potting up and keeping somewhere shaded till roots appear. It often self-seeds itself about if it's happy, but is easy enough to weed out.

## How to use

If you have a cough or cold appearing, make a tea of 1–2 teaspoons of dried leaves and flowers that have been slightly crushed and steeped in 1 cup of boiling water for 10–15 minutes. Cover the cup with a saucer, or, better still, brew a teapot so as not to lose any essential oils. This tea can be drunk up to three times a day. Make a stronger version of the tea by using 2–3 teaspoons of herb. This can then be turned into a cough syrup by adding honey to the ratio of one part tea to two parts by volume honey. It tastes heavenly.

My favourite way of using hyssop is to make a herbal syrup using raw honey. For this it's best to use fresh flowers, but dried will do.

Pack a glass jar with the flower tops and cover with raw honey. Allow to steep on a warm windowsill, the sunnier the better as this will help draw out the goodness into the honey. Leave for 2 weeks, then strain through muslin and a strainer, discarding the flowers and bottling the remaining honey. This should be taken at the first scratches of a sore throat or cough.

# LADY'S MANTLE

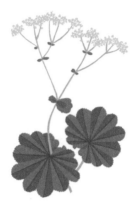

**Other Names** Garden lady's mantle, alpine lady's mantle.

**Botanical Names** *Alchemilla vulgaris, Alchemilla mollis, Alchemilla alpina.*

**Family** Rosaceae (rose family).

**Parts Used** Leaves, flower shoots.

**Plant Properties** Astringent, diuretic, anti-inflammatory, wound-healing.

**Uses** Styptic for cuts and wounds, gargle for mouth ulcers, to treat diarrhoea, menstrual problems and mastitis.

**Preparations** Poultices, teas.

**Considerations** It is very astringent, so a note of caution if you are prone to constipation.

The dewdrops on lady's mantle leaves glistening in the sun are one of the joys of the morning garden; a vase full of the tiny acid-green flowers another. Lady's mantle is the sort of plant that finds its way to your garden and then dances around as it pleases. Wanton to self-seed liberally into the smallest cracks of a path or edge of a bed, it flops about in a hopelessly romantic way and often is the plant that ties together a garden. It's a much-loved, if ubiquitous, cottage garden plant, but few know of its medicinal properties.

Lady's mantle, along with the smaller alpine lady's mantle, has a long folk history. As their name suggests they've been chiefly used for women's health, specifically to alleviate painful periods and stimulate menstrual flow. The astringent properties mean the tea is useful in the treatment of diarrhoea and can also be used as a mouthwash for sores and ulcers or as a gargle. The leaves can be used for mastitis, placed in the bra.

I've heard it said that alpine lady's mantle, *Alchemilla alpina*, with its smaller, delicate silver-edged pleated leaves, is the stronger medicinal herb. It's certainly very pretty and perfect for those with limited space as it grows to no more than 20cm high and is perfectly content in a pot, alpine trough or rock garden setting. It likes very well-drained but moist conditions (easier to replicate in a pot if your soil is far from this) and is often found growing beside streams, in meadows and on snow-bed sites in the mountains.

# How to grow

All three species will find their own place, being happy self-seeders. They like sunny, very free-draining spots and grow in thin soils. The garden lady's mantle, *Alchemilla mollis*, will tolerate some shade but tends to grow smaller and more poorly with lack of sun. If you don't want it to self-seed (and it will!), make sure you cut back the flowers before they drop their thousands of tiny black seeds. The whole plant can be cut back hard after flowering for a new flush of leaves.

Indeed, this is often necessary when the older leaves start to look tired, particularly if they have gone through a period of drought. Water well after cutting back. This plant remains blissfully free of any pest or disease.

Harvest the leaves and recently opened flowers, preferably in early morning. You can use this herb fresh or dried. A midsummer harvest should mean you get a second flush and smattering of flowers for later use.

## How to use

This is such a kind herb, and as it is safe for general use it's well worth adding to other herbal teas to bulk them out. For an infusion for period pain or menstrual issues pour 1 cup of boiling water over 2 teaspoons of crushed dried herb, or double that of chopped fresh herbs (both flowers and leaves), and infuse for 10–15 minutes, covering the contents. This can be drunk up to three times a day.

To use as an astringent for diarrhoea, or mouthwash, you need to extract the tannins from the leaves. To do this bring the leaves (same dosage as the tea) to boil for a few minutes. This mixture will make your mouth pucker and feel somewhat dry from all the tannins; gargle for a sore throat, or drink the tea for diarrhoea. It can also be an astringent for problem or oily skin. Use it as you might a toner and apply to blemishes and acne.

# LAVENDER

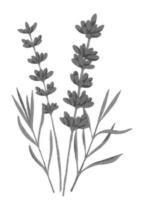

**Botanical Name** *Lavandula angustifolia.*

**Family** Lamiaceae (mint family).

**Parts Used** Flowers, buds, seeds, leaves.

**Plant Properties** Aromatic, antimicrobial, nervine, carminative.

**Uses** Antibacterial and antifungal infections, anti-inflammatory tension, aids sleep, anxiety, headaches, insect bites.

**Preparations** Culinary, infusions, strewing herb for baths, teas.

**Considerations** Do not use internally without direction from a doctor. Never use lavender from florists or garden shops that are not identified clearly as organically grown as these may contain systemic pesticides that are not approved for culinary use. Likewise, if you are doing a bit of urban foraging, don't harvest lavender that is on a busy road or growing in potentially polluted soils.

There's a bank of lavender that sprawls out from behind a fence that I pass on the way to the shops. It was planted as part of a new build housing scheme and no one has paid it a jot of attention since, so it makes the most of life by reaching on to the pavement. I have a habit of running my hand along the waving flower heads to take in its deep aroma before hitting the busy streets. On hot days you don't even need to bruise the leaves for the oil; it seems to soak into this corner of concrete and tarmac and sing with bees. I thank the inspired landscape architect every time I pass.

Lavender is a plant that calls out to be touched, begs to be stroked, minds little if you pull a bit off to roll about in your fingers. It produces its essential oils to keep off hungry herbivores that might make light work of it on a sun-bleached hillside in southern France. But our relationship to this plant is ancient and is based around our love of its smell as much as its medicinal properties. Lavender reminds us of a simple lesson: our relationship with plants is primal. We evolved in an environment thick with plants. Many of us dismiss or ignore the vegetation that surrounds us these days, but our ancestors were bound by it. I think that's why gardeners and plant enthusiasts develop such intimate relationships with their intricate worlds. For me lavender is a plant that reminds even the most jaded of that primal connection; they can't resist instinctively turning their nose to follow the waft, a reminder of who we are.

Apparently lions, tigers and jaguars are similarly fascinated by lavender's smell. Chester's zookeepers make herb pillows for big cats to play with. I realize most of you won't have a pet lion, but just in case . . .

Lavender's medicinal use can be traced back at least 2,500 years in the Mediterranean where it hails from. It was (and still is) most commonly used in bathing and laundry. It spread through northern Europe in the Middle Ages and its popularity has never died. The lavender industry is as strong today as it has ever been. Climate change poses some threats as increasingly hot and dry summers in the southern regions of France mean that the plants cannot retain enough moisture to survive over winter. An invasive insect has also appeared, transmitting a bacterial parasite that results in flowers not properly forming and a consequent reduction in essential oil. An ironic state of affairs, as the essential oils are known to be very good at keeping insects at bay. Monoculture fields of lavender may look idyllic, but they are not a diverse ecosystem and pests make light work of such easy conditions. Perhaps this is another reason to grow your own.

There are thirty-nine species of lavender, which are mainly found growing in sunny, dry regions from the Mediterranean to South East Asia and the Canary Islands. The best lavender for medicinal properties is *L. angustifolia*, which is commonly known as English or true lavender. Hybrid lavenders, such as *L. × intermedia* (a hybrid cross between *L. angustifolia* and Portuguese lavender, *L. latifolia*), often known as Lavandin, are used widely in the scent industry for their essential oil. It smells heavenly, but does not have the properties that are so useful in herbal remedies.

Lavender's heady scent is more than just sweetness; its properties help us to relax and aid sleep. For centuries sheets, pillows and baths have been scented with the flowers and seeds to aid a good night's sleep. Numerous studies show that smelling lavender reduces general anxiety and lowers levels of stress. A number of studies have also shown that lavender lowers blood pressure, heart rate and skin temperature, which might be why it aids sleep. One study showed how both lavender and rosemary essential oil reduced the level of cortisol, the stress hormone, in saliva.

Lavender has a long history for relieving pain. There's some evidence to show that inhaling lavender helps to address migraine headaches. Many beekeepers use lavender oil to relieve bee stings and reduce swelling, and massaging with essential oil is said to be effective in reducing painful periods.

In folklore lavender essential oil has long been used to treat minor burns and reduce pain and improve healing. Lavender essential oil can be used directly on the skin, but should be kept out of the eyes, nose, mouth and sensitive mucous membranes.

Lavender flowers and seeds help aid digestion and are kinder to those who can't stomach the heat of ginger. Combined with camomile, lavender makes a wonderful after-dinner tea.

# How to grow

Lavender is not long-lived so don't expect your plants to be with you forever. Neither should you expect a nice neat shape – in warm, wetter climates lavender tends to grow straggly. The simplest way around this is to cut the plant back by a third immediately after flowering as this will stimulate a flush of new growth. Lavender rarely responds well to being cut back into old wood, so if your plant is leggy, it's better to start again with a new plant or take cuttings. Semi-ripe hardwood cuttings taken in July or August will root quickly.

Lavender is incredibly drought-resistant, but growing in a pot and failing to water regularly will result in a stressed plant. *L. angustifolia* will grow up to 1 metre tall and the same width, so a tiny 30cm pot will make it unhappy. Lavenders also need full sun and any sort of shade will induce leggy growth. Potash (from wood-burning fires with no coal) will encourage flowering, but high-nitrogen fertilizers and manures will result in floppy growth. Lavender must be grown in free-draining soils; heavy clay will cause the plants to rot off in winter.

If you have limited space, then the dwarf cultivars *L. angustifolia* 'Little Lottie', 'Miss Muffet' and 'Nana Alba' (white-flowered), all grow to 30cm high and are perfect for pots, low hedges and the fronts of borders.

# How to use

## Lavender tea

Lavender tea is, as you might expect, perfumed and floral. Use 1–3g of lavender seed heads or dried flowering heads per cup of boiling water, 250ml, and allow to steep, covered, for 10 minutes. This can be taken up to three times a day.

You can use the cold tea to wash minor burns, open sores or minor skin infections where its antibacterial properties will help with healing.

## Lavender bath

Put several handfuls of seed heads, dried flowers or leaves (if no flower heads are available) in a muslin bag and run a hot bath over it. Best before bed as you're going to be sleepy.

You can also make lavender salts for the bath. Combine 1 cup of sea salt with 2 cups of Epsom salts and a handful of dried lavender seeds. Use a strainer over your plughole to catch the seeds or tie the bath-salt mixture in muslin and allow the salt to dissolve.

## Lavender sheets

Chop whole stems of lavender flower spikes with the seed heads and dry out of direct sunlight, then put sprigs of these between your laundered sheets in the airing cupboard. Not only will it keep moths at bay, when you slip into clean, lavender-scented sheets you will truly feel like an accomplished adult.

# LEMON BALM

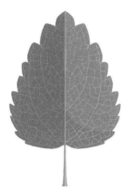

**Other Names** Common balm, balm mint.

**Botanical Name** *Melissa officinalis.*

**Family** Lamiaceae (mint family).

**Parts Used** Leaves and stems just before flowering.

**Plant Properties** Aromatic, antiviral, relaxing, improves digestion, diaphoretic, carminative, sedative, antispasmodic.

**Uses** Digestion, coughs, anxiety, nervousness, stress, viral infections, insect bites, stings.

**Preparations** Culinary, infusions, strewing herb for baths, teas.

**Considerations** There is evidence to show that lemon balm may inhibit thyroid functions, particularly for an underactive thyroid condition. Consult your doctor or herbalist.

We should listen to the bees more often, for if you have a patch or a pot of lemon balm in flower it will soon be covered with all manner of bees, from hairy bumbles to honeybees, and they clearly know a thing or two about how wonderful lemon balm is — this humble herb is a powerful, yet gentle medicine. The Latin name

*Melissa* references this; Melissa (*mel* meaning honey in Greek) in Greek mythology was a nymph who understood the wisdom of the bees and knew how to collect honey. *Melissa* has long been in cultivation in its native Mediterranean but it was introduced as a medicine by the Arabs who used it as a sedative or tonic tea. I think it might be one of my most favourite herbs.

Lemon balm is known for its calming and soothing properties, be that for a restless sleeper, an upset stomach or just the tired, frayed nerves of a long week. It's safe enough to give to children and is best drunk as a tea, where its gentle mild flavour seems to be liked by everyone. This is excellent before bed, particularly for the restless sort who toss and turn. One study showed that, when combined with valerian, lemon balm supported healthy sleep cycles in menopausal women. It has very high antioxidant levels and is said to reduce DNA damage and its antiviral properties have been used for herpes and cold sores.*

## How to grow

Lemon balm is incredibly easy to grow, and is happy in sun or part shade, in a pot or in the ground. It is fairly drought-tolerant, but if you're growing it in a pot it's best not to stress it out and to water

* S. Taavoni, N. Nazem Ekbatani and H. Haghani, 'Valerian/Lemon Balm Use for Sleep Disorders During Menopause' (*Complementary Therapies in Clinical Practice*, 19(4), 2013), pp. 193–6. https://doi.org/10.1016/j.ctcp.2013.07.002 [Accessed 21 January 2019]

A. Zeraatpishe et. al., 'Effects of *Melissa officinalis* L. on Oxidative Status and DNA Damage in Subjects Exposed to Long-term Low-dose Ionizing Radiation' (*Toxicology and Industrial Health*, 27(3), 2010), pp. 205–212. https://doi.org/10.1177/0748233710383889 [Accessed 21 January 2019]

regularly through hot periods. Use a pot at least 30cm in diameter or bigger so that it has space to grow. It will self-seed, so if you don't want it moving about, chop back the stems after flowering to the new growth below and water well; this will also give you a new flourish of leaves to pick. There are several varieties, including variegated and golden versions, such as 'Aurea'. Lemon balm essential oil is not common and very expensive to produce because it has such tiny amounts in its leaves; seven tonnes of plant material is needed to produce just one kilogram of oil. 'Quedlinburger Niederliegende' is a variety bred for such production as it has a higher essential oil content (which is around 0.1 per cent, comprising eugenol, tannins, terpenes, as well as rosmarinic acid, which is one of its most important active components). 'Compacta' is a dwarf variety that only grows to 15cm high (as opposed to the 80cm of the straight species) and therefore is good for pots and window boxes. There's also a delicious lime balm, *M. officinalis* 'Lime Balm', that smells distinctly, as you'd expect, of lime.

When grown in the ground, lemon balm is clump-forming with spreading rhizomes and it will take over smaller, more delicate plants. However, it is very easy to keep in check: just slice off chunks of the plant with a sharp spade. It will readily self-seed if you don't deadhead it, and it can become invasive.

Named varieties of lemon balm should be bought, but the species can be sown on a warm windowsill or in a heated propagator. It may take up to three weeks to germinate, at which point pot on into individual containers and plant out when all threat of frost has passed.

# How to use

It is possible to dry lemon balm, but as it is in growth for nearly all but the worst of winter, you can almost always find a few leaves to pick. If you do dry it, do so in small quantities so that you are just using it for the few months when it is not bountiful, because it certainly loses its flavour and some of its oomph when dried.

I eat a lot of lemon balm. On its own the slightly hairy leaves are not that appealing, though a few in salads are acceptable, but I find it makes an excellent base for green sauces and salsas. Its mild flavour is the perfect starting point for adding more bitter herbs, such as dandelion leaves, or stronger flavours, such as mint or coriander.

## Lemon balm tea

Lemon balm can be consumed regularly (as long as you don't have a thyroid condition), particularly as a tea. For a light infusion try a teaspoon of leaves; for a stronger brew you can increase this to 4–6g infused for 10 minutes. This can be taken morning and evening or when needed. This is my go-to tea for an upset stomach, if I am a little hungover or just need a quiet break from the world.

## Lemon balm tea for a good night's sleep

2 parts lemon balm
1 part lavender
2 parts oat straw
1 cup water

Combine the ingredients and pour over 1 cup of boiling water and infuse in a covered container or teapot for 10–15 minutes. Drink before bed.

## A floral lemon balm tea

750ml water

½ cup lemon balm

4–5 lemon verbena leaves

2 tablespoons rose petals

Add 750ml of just boiled water to the herbs and allow to steep for 4 hours or overnight. Strain and add honey if desired. Gently reheat or drink iced. Drink within 24 hours.

## Lemon balm sun tea

2 or 3 sprigs lemon balm,
   gently bruised
   (or 1 tablespoon dried leaves)

1 slice lemon

500ml water

Combine ingredients and water and leave a 1-litre glass jar or jug in the sun for roughly 4 hours. You may wish to cover the opening with muslin to keep insects out; the sun will gently brew the leaves, creating a mild, refreshing drink. If there's no sun around, you can use lukewarm boiled water instead.

## Lemon balm bath

If your plants are doing particularly well and you find yourself with an excess of lemon balm, pick armfuls for the bath, let the water turn a pleasant light green and enjoy this incredibly soothing bath at the end of a long and tiring day.

## Lemon balm oil

Prepare a herbal oil of lemon balm by infusing crushed and bruised leaves in an oil that won't go off quickly, such as olive or jojoba. Fill a jar with leaves that are clean but completely dry, and then fill with oil. Stir the mixture well and then leave for 2 weeks, before straining and using the oil as desired. It is good to use as a salve for sore lips, particularly cold sores. The oil should be used up within 3 weeks or stored in the fridge.

# LEMON VERBENA

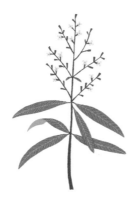

**Botanical Name** *Aloysia citrodora.*
**Family** Verbenaceae (verbena family).
**Parts Used** Leaves, flowers.

**Plant Properties** Aromatic.
**Uses** Flavouring.
**Preparations** Cordials, culinary, teas.
**Considerations** None known.

Lemon verbena hails all the way from South America and was brought to Europe by Spanish and Portuguese explorers in the seventeenth century, when there was a fever for new plants and flavours, and botanic gardens were packed with strange exotics. It was quickly cultivated for its oil, which is rich in citral that is, as its name suggests, reminiscent of lemon; the leaves when bruised instantly smell like boiled lemon sweets. Lemon verbena is included in this book because of its nostalgic scent alone; for if it has any herbal properties no one has bothered to say much of them. It can be used in puddings, jams, salad dressings, Greek yoghurt, countless beverages (try a few leaves instead of lemon in a gin and tonic), or you can stuff it under the skin of a roasting chicken or use it in a sauce for fish, create a flavoured butter, combine with coconut for puddings and curries or use as a substitute for lemongrass, and that is to say nothing of what it will do when you pour hot water on it.

Lemon verbena is an excellent tisane, delicious, light, sour enough to make after dinner, sweet enough to ease the morning routine and perfect for every hour in between. Lemon verbena also adds a fresh, sweet note to those herbs that can, frankly, start tasting uniformly grassy, straw-like, bitter or dull.

# How to grow

Lemon verbena is a shrub and can grow easily to 1.5 metres tall with woody stems. However, it is not hardy, and only in the most sheltered, sunny gardens can it be planted out to grow as it pleases. You can often buy small plug plants that will need to be potted up immediately. Pot this up regularly; the bigger it grows, the hardier it gets. It should be grown in full sun and although it can tolerate drought, it flourishes when watered at least once a week during the hot summer months so that its soil is moist but not soggy.

Lemon verbena should be pruned back to half its size in autumn. At this point you will probably prune off many a healthy leaf; do not waste these – they dry quickly and keep their flavour if stored in an airtight container. You can use them all winter long until the new leaves appear. Potted lemon verbena needs to overwinter somewhere sheltered and frost-free. It certainly won't like a centrally heated house, which will just prompt it to start growing again, but weakly, which nearly always results in the plant being covered in aphids.

Instead, tuck it into the lea of the house and cover with a little fleece until spring comes back round.

# How to use

## Lemon verbena tisane

Two or three leaves in a cup of boiling water makes an excellent tisane for any time of the day. It is the perfect flavouring to other herbal teas, working well with lemon balm, thyme, rose petals and camomile, and is often the flavouring needed to persuade those disdainful of herbal tea.

# LEMONGRASS

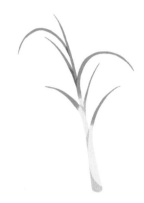

**Botanical Name** *Cymbopogon citratus.*
**Family** Poaceae (grass family).
**Parts Used** Stems, leaves.
**Plant Properties** Aromatic, antispasmodic, stomach-soothing, astringent, antimicrobial, antifungal, improves digestion, nervine, mild sedative, anti-inflammatory.
**Uses** Digestion, coughs, antifungal, antibacterial, insect bites, aids sleep, skin tonic.
**Preparations** Culinary, infusions, strewing herb for baths, teas.
**Considerations** None known.

Lemongrass is a tropical grass from South Asia that loves wet, hot conditions. It's quite possible to grow it in the UK, but it has to come indoors for the winter and will rarely get to its full height in our mild summers. You're unlikely to yield fat stems to cook with; however, in my experience, home-grown lemongrass packs a stronger punch than anything bought from the shops so what you don't get in size, you get in flavour.

My best tip for lemongrass is to put a piece from the supermarket in a glass of water until you see roots a couple of centimetres long. Be patient; it can take weeks. Once they appear transplant into compost with a little added grit. Lemongrass loves wet conditions and is often found growing in damp and wet spots in the tropics, but it doesn't, I find, like sitting in a slump of poorly drained soil, hence the grit. I make sure the plant sits in a little water for part of the day (it doesn't like anaerobic conditions, so if it's sitting in water, remove the saucer, drain it away and replace). If this sounds like a lot of work, keep it by the kitchen sink and slosh clean water over it when you do the washing up. In the summer you can take it outside for a little holiday; it thrives in bright, sunny conditions and will put on considerable growth.

# How to use

## Lemongrass tea
Lemongrass tea does taste like its eponymous lemon but with a distinct sweetness and without significant tartness. It's great on its own or mixed with other, less flavoursome herbs. Lemongrass can be added to other sleep-inducing teas, such as oat, lemon balm or lime blossom tea. It can also be added to any tea to aid digestion. It's particularly good after dinner with a lemon balm and lemon verbena mix in equal parts.

## For culinary use
Lemongrass is widely used in South Asian cooking to flavour dishes. It works particularly well in savoury dishes with chicken, coconut

milk and seafood and in broths, but shouldn't be ignored for sweet dishes. Consider adding to panna cotta, ice cream or sweet coconut puddings. Lemongrass pairs well with both pear and rhubarb.

## For medicinal use

Lemongrass has long been used in Brazilian traditional folk medicine to treat gastric disturbances. Recent small-scale scientific studies suggest that it might have gastroprotective properties against gastric ulcers, though the tests were conducted on mice.*

When drunk in tea, lemongrass's antimicrobial and anti-inflammatory properties can eliminate fungal infections and help with stomach issues. Steep 1 or 2 teaspoons of chopped lemongrass stalks in a cup of boiling water and cover for 10–12 minutes. Drink up to three times a day.

Due to its delicious smell and its antimicrobial qualities lemongrass makes a great skin tonic and is used widely in the beauty industry. Use the tea cooled as a toner. Alternatively add handfuls of lemongrass leaves to a bath for a refreshing soak. I especially like the combination of dried rose petals and lemongrass.

* C., Fernandes et al., 'Investigation of the Mechanisms Underlying the Gastroprotective Effect of *Cymbopogon citratus* Essential Oil' (*Journal of Young Pharmacists*, 4(1), 2012), pp. 28–32. https://www.ncbi.nlm.nih.gov/pmc/articles/PMC3326778/ [Accessed 22 January 2019]

# LIME BLOSSOM

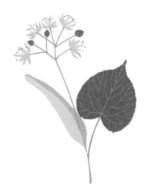

**Other Name** Linden, little-leafed lime.

**Botanical Name** *Tilia cordata*. (Both *Tilia americana* and *Tilia platyphyllos* can be substituted for *T. cordata*.)

**Family** Malvaceae (mallow family).

**Parts Used** Young leaves, flowers in the early-flowering stage.

**Plant Properties** Nervine, antispasmodic, hypotensive, diuretic, anti-inflammatory, diaphoretic, astringent.

**Uses** Relaxant, migraines, colds and flu, aids sleep.

**Preparations** Culinary, teas.

**Considerations** The pollen may cause hay fever and allergic reactions in some individuals.

When Proust wrote of madeleines dipped in tea he made famous the journey of memory, that 'Proustian moment' we all have when something involuntarily evokes the past so strongly that just the mere whiff of a baked madeleine can take you home. But all that hype about Proust's madeleine should really be about lime flowers. Proust was dipping his cake into linden tea and it's the tea that actually evokes his past, his aunt's garden filled with flowers.

Lime blossom, or linden, tea is delicious, honeyed and distinct in aroma and flavour. I can't drink the stuff and stay awake, so its famed relaxant effect clearly works well on me. Lime blossom's antispasmodic properties are said to be very good for those who suffer from leg cramps at night. Lime blossom tea is also used to soothe teething children, and it is thought to be helpful for lowering cholesterol and act as a remedy for nervous tension.

I don't have the space to grow a tree that large – it easily reaches 30 metres tall – but my park, thanks to my local beekeepers who have hives there, is full of the trees and therefore all I have to do in early June is go and harvest the flowers and dry them quickly somewhere cool and dark.

The leaves are delicious when young, soft and lime-green and a perfectly good substitute for lettuce; in fact, I'd say a better one because they never go soggy in a sandwich.

## How to grow

The tree is easy enough to grow from seed, but you might wait a long while to harvest enough flowers. This is a common tree in parks, often found around housing developments and other amenity areas. You'll know when it's out because you'll hear the bees buzzing with delight and smell the strong, sweet honey scent from the other side of the road.

The leaves are rounded to heart-shaped, deciduous and alternately arranged. The flowers are small, yellow-green and produced in clusters of five to eleven. The flowers should be picked at early maturity. The young leaves are most prevalent in spring and early summer.

# How to use

The flowers should be picked not long after opening, when headiest in scent, and should be dried promptly out of direct sunlight. They are highly susceptible to both moisture and sunlight and should be stored when dry in an airtight container somewhere cool and dark.

## Lime blossom tea

Lime blossom tea is made from the crushed dried flowers. Steep a heaped teaspoon (1g) for 5 minutes in 1 cup of hot water, then strain. The tea will make most people sweat, so it's useful for the beginning of a cold or flu. Drink the tea, go to bed and then drink more fluids when you wake up and you can often nip the earliest signs of such a virus in the bud. For a cooling drink, try sweetening the tea with honey before refrigerating, then pouring over ice. Dip madeleines in if you so desire. Lime blossom tea has also been used to flavour confectionary, cakes and bread.

## For medicinal use

You can add a handful of flowers in a muslin bag to a bath for a relaxing soak. It is said to calm the overstimulated and aid a rapid, dreamless sleep.

Make a poultice of fresh lime leaves, mashed and muddled with a little water, to treat wounds, sprains and swellings, where the astringent nature and healing mucilage in the leaves is said to do wonders.

Honey from the lime tree is delicious and reputed to have medicinal properties that are good for colds and sore throats.

# LOVAGE

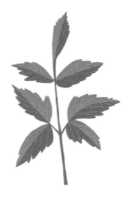

**Botanical Name** *Levisticum officinalis.*
**Family** Apiaceae (carrot family).
**Parts Used** Leaves, stems, roots, seeds.

**Plant Properties** Aromatic, stimulant, carminative.
**Uses** Digestion, anti-flatulence.
**Preparations** Culinary, teas.

**It is recommended that strong tea from the roots or seeds is avoided during pregnancy. Prolonged usage or dosage of lovage can cause photosensitivity in some people. Avoid large doses if you have issues with your kidneys and consult a doctor or registered herbalist.**

Lovage is the giant cousin to parsley and celery, having a note of both, but sweeter with a touch of cumin. It can grow to 2 metres tall and its roots run deep, so remember this when you buy that tiny 9cm pot. It needs space, but it is rather unfussy about its quality. Its deep taproots mean it can mine all sorts of exciting nutrients and minerals in the soil that are not available to shallower-rooted types and allow it to grow in rather poor conditions.

Once upon a time lovage was popular for both medicinal and culinary purposes; it flavoured soup, stews and liqueurs. Today it's the secret ingredient of Jägermeister and is also used in gin and vodka. Lovage works much like a stock cube without the salt, its celery/parsley notes adding a depth to cooking that we now substitute with celery. The cool, crunchy stems of the celery as we know it is a fairly modern taste, needing vast quantities of water to grow as it does. Before celery, lovage was what people reached for. Its leaves were used in salads. The roots were peeled, cooked and often candied to be used as a gentle stimulant to keep people awake during long church services. Cordials were made with the seed, often along with yarrow and tansy.

Historically lovage was also proffered for all number of medicinal issues. The kidneys, stomach and the cardiovascular, lymphatic and reproductive systems are all gently stimulated by lovage and traditionally it has been used for thousands of years for digestion and flatulence, often by chewing the seeds.

The long, deep taproot absorbs salt from the soil, so consequently lovage leaves and roots have a high salt content that has been used to drain mild oedema (excess water fluid in cells, tissues or body cavities) as well as conditions like gout, arthritis and bladder and kidney stones.

## How to grow

Lovage is erratic from seed; usually only half will germinate and therefore it's worth sowing double what you need. You usually only need one plant in most gardens. Seed should be sown fresh in the autumn or spring and the young seedlings overwintered somewhere sheltered from direct frost until they can be planted out the following spring.

If you know someone who already has a plant, you can split or divide the root ball. Do this in spring and make sure you get a section with both a growing tip and root. Plant out in a good fertile position. It is possible to grow lovage permanently in a pot or container, but it does need to be big; a half-barrel is ideal. It will need regular watering, although lovage is surprisingly drought-tolerant and a tough thing. Kept in too small a pot, lovage will be very unhappy, often turning yellowish and stunted.

# How to use

Harvest the leaves before flowering, and the root and seeds in autumn. Chop the root up before drying, because once it is desiccated it's rather hard work.

## Lovage tea

Simmer in a covered pot 1–2 tablespoons of chopped dried lovage root in 1 cup of water for 5 minutes and then let it rest, still covered, for 10 minutes. This can be drunk up to three times a day.

Infusing the leaves in water overnight will make a refreshing drink that can be drunk up to three times a day. Use 4–5 tablespoons of fresh leaves in 1 litre of water.

You can also make a tea out of the dried leaves. Use 1 tablespoon of chopped dried leaves in 1 pint of water, steeped for 10 minutes. This can be drunk up to three times a day.

In theory there is nothing to stop you (unless pregnant) drinking all three methods three times a day. But be sensible – choose one and stick to that.

## For culinary use

More often than not, what is labelled as celery salt actually contains lovage. Use dried seeds and blend in a coffee grinder or mortar and pestle with sea salt to taste. First grind the seeds, taste, and then start adding small quantities of salt to taste. Go slowly on adding the salt because the seed is naturally salty in flavour. The seed can also be used in pickling mixtures, breads or in savoury biscuits to go with cheese.

You can use the leaves in salads, soups, stews and anywhere you might celery. They are considerably stronger in flavour than shop-bought celery so use sparingly. Lovage's hollow stem is excellent in a Bloody Mary. For the ultimate Bloody Mary, my friend, the brilliant gardener and cook Mark Diacono, recommends steeping lovage leaves in a bottle of vodka for several weeks and then straining.

The stems and the roots can be candied the same way you would angelica. You can also cook the stems, peeled, like you might salsify.

# MACE,

## *see* YARROW

---

# MALLOWS

**Botanical Names** *Malva sylvestris, Malva verticillata* 'Crispa', *Malva neglecta, Althaea officinalis, Alcea rosea.*

**Family** Malvaceae (mallow family).

**Parts Used** All parts of the plant, in particular leaves, flowers, roots.

**Plant Properties** Astringent, demulcent, diuretic, emollient, expectorant, laxative.

**Uses** Bruises, inflammations, insect bites; the roots and leaves are used for the treatment of the respiratory system.

**Preparations** Culinary, infusions, salves, teas.

**Considerations** The roots of *A. officinalis* are particularly mucilaginous and may interfere with the absorption of other drugs.

All mallows are largely interchangeable as far as their medicinal properties go. However, the marshmallow, *Althaea officinalis,* has far superior roots, decoctions of which can be used to treat inflamed mucous membranes, a rasping throat from a dry cough, and upper respiratory or urinary tract infections. The marshmallow is a handsome plant and well worth growing for that reason alone, but for good roots you need damp, fertile ground like that at the edge of a large pond and that's perhaps trickier for the average back garden. Still, if you find yourself with a large pond or damp spot, then this is your plant.

Although the roots provide gentle, yet powerful medicine, the leaves and flowers shouldn't be ignored. For that matter all the other mallows – common, *M. sylvestris*; vegetable or Chinese mallow, *M. verticillata* 'Crispa'; dwarf, *M. neglecta*; and even the common hollyhock – have aerial parts that can be used.

Without doubt the vegetable mallow from China is the best to eat. The soft, slightly chewy leaves make them an excellent salad addition, but they can also be cooked like spinach. The leaves chopped into scrambled eggs for breakfast are quite something, like spinach but with a better texture. All mallow leaves are rounded with five to seven lobes, but the crinkled edges of *M. verticillata* 'Crispa' make it highly attractive and it will happily self-seed around your garden, so it is a very low-maintenance edible. And unlike spinach it won't be bothered by slugs and won't bolt to flower at the first mention of heat. It's a better-tasting, lazier version with more health benefits. It should be the new spinach.

The common mallow, *M. sylvestris*, and dwarf mallow, *M. neglecta*, have a wide geographical distribution from Europe to Asia and into North America. They grow mostly as weeds, and are easy enough to forage for, but stay away from polluted soil or those that are too nitrogen-rich. You often find them on old manure heaps; well-rotted manure is no issue, but you shouldn't eat too many leaves off plants growing in fresh or recent manure because the plant concentrates too many nitrates into the leaves and too much nitrate in the diet can be toxic, though you would have to eat an awful lot every day for a prolonged period to suffer any adverse effects.

The garden hollyhock, another member of the mallow family, has slightly tougher leaves that I'd avoid eating unless desperately hungry for such things, though the leaves are perfectly good to use in tea. However, as the garden hollyhock is so susceptible to hollyhock rust – small, bright yellow and orange pustules that appear on the upper sides of the leaves – the plants may be sprayed with fungicides to prevent this from happening and you do not want to go anywhere near those leaves, so don't assume a garden centre plant is suitable for edible or medicinal properties. You also shouldn't use leaves infected with rust; the plant is not in good health and should be left alone. I've given up growing hollyhocks in my garden for this reason, but I find the vegetable mallow is somewhat immune to the rust.

Marshmallow roots, as the name suggests, were the original ingredient in marshmallow sweets, which were used as medicine as much as being toasted on the fire. The soft, mucilaginous nature of the root was employed as a confectionary cough sweet. You can't just chew the roots raw, though; they have to be boiled and processed first. The roots of the other mallows are woodier and therefore are rarely used for medicinal or culinary purposes. However, both common and dwarf mallows have been foraged for use as an egg substitute. When boiled in water the roots quickly thicken, and as long as you have the right ratio of root to liquid (the roots should only just be covered) then you can whisk this thickened water, removing the roots first, into a scrambled-egg-like substance. This occurs because the mucilage, a complex blend of carbohydrate, proteins and sugar, is used by the plant to hold on to water and as the roots are essentially a storage organ it makes sense that it is packed with the stuff. This watery mixture has been used as a meringue substitute and tastes about as interesting as egg whites, which is to say quite bland. However, mallow root can be a useful vegan substitute for egg.

Woodier mallow roots were traditionally dried and frayed, then used as a toothbrush, again utilizing the mucilaginous properties to help with gum infections and mouth ulcers. There is some evidence to show that, taken in high quantities, these properties might interfere with how other medicines are absorbed, so be aware of this if you decide to experiment with the root.

# How to grow

Marshmallow, *A. officinalis*, is a native herbaceous perennial that has soft, hairy, grey-green rounded leaves and stems and small clusters of saucer-shaped white to palest lilac-pink flowers that appear from midsummer to early autumn.

Although it will tolerate a wide range of conditions, marshmallow does grow best in fertile, rich, very moist, but not boggy conditions in full sun. This is essential if you want a decent harvest of roots. It is possible to grow the plant in a very large pot (50 litres plus) if these conditions are hard to replicate in the ground. You will have to water the pot daily in the summer. In autumn the whole plant can be cut back down or left standing over winter for insect habitat. Seed should be sown in midsummer and young plants overwintered in a cold frame to be planted out the following spring. It grows up to 2.5 metres tall and 1–1.5 metres in spread.

The common mallow, *M. sylvestris*, is a perennial herbaceous native that grows wild in many locations in the UK, most prolifically in the south of England, though it can be found in many urban areas, alongside motorways and in grassy verges. The seed should be sown in late spring and it prefers full sun. It grows in a wide variety of soils but prefers free-draining conditions. It grows up to 1.5 metres tall and the same in width, though many of the wild plants you might find will be considerably smaller. It's not something I'd necessarily grow in my garden, too weedy, though I'd be very happy to forage it if I found it appearing naturally.

Both the vegetable mallow, *M. verticillata* 'Crispa', and the dwarf mallow, *M. neglecta*, are annual or short-lived biennials. The dwarf mallow is a treasure to find when foraging, but perhaps too weedy for the garden for most tastes. The vegetable mallow, however, is a true gourmand delight and a worthy addition to any garden. The seeds for both should be sown from late spring to midsummer. Both plants will self-seed and tend to prefer fertile positions in sun to part shade.

# How to use

The leaves of *M. sylvestris*, *M. neglecta* and *M. verticillata* should be picked when young and tender for eating.

## For medicinal use

The leaves of any species, if healthy, can be lightly steamed and used as an application to swellings, infections and chapped or dry skin. The roots of any species can also be mashed up raw and blended with water to make a cooling poultice for treating minor burns or new wounds. The roots of *A. officinalis*, marshmallow, can be boiled until tender and then mashed up and applied, hot but not boiling, between layers of muslin to swellings, puncture wounds, infected wounds and difficult splinters.

You can make a tea or a cold infusion of leaves and flowers, either fresh or dried (the latter in winter, as there's unlikely to be any fresh around). The tea is bland-tasting, but kind to sore throats, and you can mix the fresh or dried leaves with other herbs such as rosemary. The dried flowers of *M. sylvestris* and *A. officinalis* (both *M. neglecta* and *M. verticillata* 'Crispa' have flowers too small to be worth processing) make a very soothing and pleasant tea.

You can add a handful of the leaves of any mallow to the bath to help with dry skin. It works nicely with oats for making a soothing bath.

Mallow roots are used to soothe irritated mucous membranes and boost the immune system. The roots of *A. officinalis* have a long use of being boiled with honey (and sometimes water). Wash young roots and slice thinly. Cover with 3 tablespoons of honey and bring quickly to the boil, so that the honey froths, then remove from the heat and allow to cool. This recipe is best made up fresh when needed rather than stored. The honeyed roots are eaten to soothe sore throats and aid with colds and chest infections. Other recipes call for adding water, using sugar rather than honey and mashing the root and rolling into balls. These are all variations on the original marsh-mallow recipe.

The raw roots of *A. officinalis* can also be chewed slowly or sucked to help with mouth ulcers.

# MARIGOLD

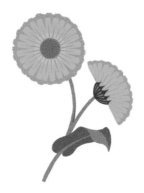

**Other Names** Pot marigold, English marigold, common marigold.

**Botanical Name** *Calendula officinalis*.

**Family** Asteraceae (sunflower or daisy family).

**Parts Used** Flowers, in particular the petals.

**Plant Properties** Antibacterial, anti-inflammatory, antiviral, antifungal.

**Uses** Soothes minor burns, cuts or irritated skin; also used to soothe the gut/digestive tract.

**Preparations** Culinary, infusions, oils, salves, teas.

**Considerations** You can overdose on calendula tea and this may cause stomach upsets or nausea.

Summer isn't summer and a garden isn't complete unless it has some *Calendula officinalis*. The radiant, brilliant orange and yellow ray petals of these flowers are like sunshine on the ground. Their resilience and easy-going nature means that I've found tattered plants flowering under a blanket of snow or bravely jollying up a tired winter with one solitary bloom waving away. To some this irrepressible nature, the endless cheerfulness of such a positive bloomer is a little too much; that and their ubiquitous nature means that they sometimes fall foul of snobbishness: 'Oh, that old thing.' Perhaps it should be one of life's lessons to gently back away from anyone who turns their nose up at a calendula. Life needs more kindness and this flower is the botanical world's offering.

The humble marigold has a history that winds right the way back to ancient Greece, where its reputation as a plant that will help you out began. Garlands of flowers were often used in ritual and religious ceremonies in Greece, Rome, India and later in Christian services, where it was referred to as Mary's gold.

Chiefly calendula is known for its skin-healing attributes, having gentle but powerful antibacterial and anti-inflammatory properties. It calms angry skin, softens dry skin, helps minor wounds heal and is mild enough to use on babies' bottoms.

The petals have a long history for culinary use, often being used as a saffron substitute, more as a dye than for flavour. There have been plenty of cheese, rice and milky puddings dyed a neon orange from the petals. I urge anyone needing a little light in their life to make a cauliflower or macaroni cheese brilliant orange with the addition of a handful of petals to the cheese sauce; there's no need to strain them out.

If I have a surplus of flowers, and that's entirely possible with even just a few plants, then I dry the petals and add them to oats for muesli and porridge. Orange sprinkles at breakfast brighten even the greyest of mornings. Likewise, the dried petals can be added to any number of teas, where they will impart their gentle anti-inflammatory and antibacterial properties. I spend the best part of summer drying flower heads (there's no need to separate the petals from the centre of the flower head) for tea as I use calendula as my main bulking agent for other herbs.

# How to grow

*C. officinalis* is a very short-lived perennial that is often grown as an annual. It can survive through frosts if it's in a sheltered enough place that receives winter sun. Temperature extremes, either very cold winters or very hot summers, will see its life shortened and it tends to only be perennial in mild climates. It will grow in any number of soil conditions, minding not one bit thin, poor soil, but it grows most lush in fertile conditions in sun or part shade. It is an important food source for a number of moths and is often prioritized by pollinators for both pollen and nectar.

*C. officinalis* is native to southern Europe, not the UK, but has been grown here for such a long time (there are references to it from the Middle Ages) that it has become widely naturalized. Its long history of cultivation has resulted in many cultivars, some with redder petals, the palest creams, apricots, rolled petals, doubles, semi-doubles or pom-poms. The natural colour range of *C. officinalis* runs from bright yellow through to deep orange, and although the many cultivars offer up some delights, I think that growing the straight species and allowing it to throw up its own bouquet of yellows and oranges is perfection enough. The straight species is also best for nectar and pollen production for beneficial insects.

Deadheading will encourage more flowers as the plant will desperately try again to produce seed, but it's not necessary; calendula's zest for life is sealed in its DNA. It rarely suffers from pests; the leaves and stem are quite sticky, which deters most sap-sucking insects, such as aphids, and once established the plants are pretty slug-repellent. Deer and rabbits will nibble at them, though.

When choosing your calendula look for a plant that exudes a dark sticky resin when the flowers are picked. Your fingers will quickly become stained and sticky. Both orange and yellow, doubles and single flowers can be rich in this resin, so don't feel you have to stick to orange petals.

# How to use

The ray sepals (the outer petals rather than the hard middle) can be used fresh or dried and added to muesli, porridge or baked goods. To dry, collect the flowers when they are fully out and place them upside down on a tray somewhere warm, preferably in the sun. The flowers will wilt rapidly and, more importantly, all the bugs and pollen beetles will make a quick retreat. After an hour, remove the flowers from the tray and shake the tray to ensure most of the pollen beetles have gone. Now remove the outer petals if you want just these for cooking or dry the flowers whole and scatter across a clean, dry tea towel. They will take a day or so to completely dry. To preserve the colour move out of direct sun.

## Calendula tea

You can make an infusion by pouring 1 cup of hot water (250ml) over 1–2 teaspoons of dried flowers and infusing for 10–15 minutes. This can be drunk up to three times a day. However, some are quite sensitive to this tea and it can cause stomach upsets and nausea; if so, don't drink any more! For most this tea has a calming anti-inflammatory action in the digestive system.

## Calendula flower oil for the skin

Calendula is antibacterial and therefore good for minor cuts, scrapes and wounds, as well as sunburn, chapped or dry skin, nappy rash and as a soothing ointment for the sore nipples of breastfeeding mums. There are numerous ways to extract the plant's antibacterial properties, usually with heat. The simplest method, however, is the folk one, using the sun, known as cold infusion or the sun method. This will store for up to a year in a cool, dark place, but don't use it if the oil smells rancid.

Dried calendula flower heads
Oil. You can use olive,
   sunflower, sweet almond,
   grapeseed, apricot or jojoba
depending on what you prefer. I tend to use sweet almond oil and jojoba.

Firstly the jar must be sterilized. Half fill your jar with dried calendula flower heads and then cover with oil to just below the top of the jar. Gently shake from side to side to remove any large air bubbles. With a clean spoon press down any petals that have floated to the top as these will become exposed to the air and may go mouldy, ruining the oil.

Seal the jar. Leave it in a sunny spot for 4 weeks (6 weeks if cloudy), after which the herbs can be strained out through a muslin-lined sieve. You can add a new batch of dried petals if you want to make a stronger oil and infuse for another 4 weeks. Strain again. Store in a sterilized jar, and seal, label and date.

You can use fresh flowers, but because of the higher water content you'll find you get quite a lot of residue and gunk that separates from the oil. If this happens you will have to strain, and this needs to be done regularly. You'll also have to double up the quantity of flower heads if you use them fresh. In my experience drying the flower heads first makes the whole thing much easier.

# MARJORAM

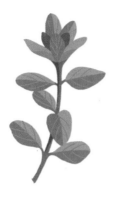

**Other Name** Sweet marjoram.
**Botanical Name** *Oregano marjorana.*
**Family** Lamiaceae (mint family).
**Parts Used** Leaves.
**Plant Properties** Improves digestion, appetite-stimulant, carminative, antimicrobial, antifungal, antibacterial, antiviral, antispasmodic, increases saliva, anti-inflammatory.
**Uses** Relieves nausea, improves appetite, calming, soothes stomach cramps, and relieves diarrhoea, constipation and the common cold.
**Preparations** Culinary, teas.
**Considerations** None known.

Marjoram, *Oregano marjorana,* is the sweet sister of oregano, *Origanum vulgare,* whose bitter, spicy, somewhat tongue-numbing flavour is known for its pairing with tomatoes for sauce. Sweet marjoram has prominent sweet pine and citrus flavours and is altogether milder than its pizza-loving sibling. Like oregano, marjoram's flavour changes and becomes more pronounced when dried and sweet marjoram is often used in zaatar and *herbes de Provence.*

Fresh, it is mild enough to be chopped into salads, used as a garnish or added at the very end of a cooked dish to preserve its flavours.

Marjoram flowers are much loved by bees and pollinators, and this is reason enough to have it in your garden. If you have enough plants, use the flowers in teas, infused waters and as a garnish for salads, though for the latter they are best removed from the woody stalks.

As a medicinal herb it is chiefly used for its antimicrobial properties and is therefore a useful ingredient in teas for colds and flu, as well as aiding digestion and helping relieve gas and stomach cramps. It can also be drunk to relieve diarrhoea and constipation, due to its having a gentle effect on the digestive system, helping to stimulate and soothe.

Oregano, *Origanum vulgare*, Greek oregano, *O. vulgarum* subsp. *hirtum*, and Syrian oregano, *O. syriacum*, can all be used interchangeably for culinary and medicinal uses.

# How to grow

Marjoram, *O. marjorana*, is a short-growing perennial found throughout Europe and into the Middle East. It is sensitive to cold, so won't always survive harsh winters, particularly if it is growing on heavy clay soil. In such conditions it should be grown as an annual. It prefers to grow in free-draining conditions in full sun, though it will tolerate some shade. After flowering it can be cut back hard to ground level for a new flush of leaves. It will self-seed with abandon, particularly along path edges. It can be propagated by seed sown in spring or by division.

Oregano, *O. vulgare*, is slightly taller than sweet marjoram, growing to 20–80cm tall. In colder climates it may have to be grown as an annual, though in the UK it is hardy. It prefers free-draining soil in a hot, sunny spot, but can thrive in a variety of locations. There are numerous cultivars, such as golden oregano, *O. vulgare* 'Aureum', which has golden foliage and a milder taste, but when grown in the shade it will revert to green shades.

*O. vulgare* subsp. *hirtum* 'Kaliteri' is a landrace from Greece (*kaliteri* means 'the best') and has particularly good flavour and pungency, and is much prized for medicinal use. It will need to be grown in full sun in very free-draining conditions.

Sicilian or Italian oregano, *O. × majoricum*, are hybrids between sweet marjoram, *O. marjorana*, and the southern Adriatic subspecies *O. vulgare* subsp. *hirtum*. They combine the best of both parents, being sweet and spicy, and work particularly well in tomato sauces.

## How to use

Use fresh as a garnish or dry. If drying, then try to cut the stems before flower buds appear. Dry somewhere cool and out of direct sunlight. You can dry on a clean pillowcase or tea towel if necessary, shaking every day to aerate the leaves. Once dry you can crumble the leaves into an airtight container and keep out of direct sunlight. Dry small batches to take you through the winter, but don't store for more than 6 months as the flavour starts to dull.

## Marjoram tea

You can use fresh or dried chopped leaves for tea. In both cases for the best flavour bring the leaves to a simmer for 10 minutes, using 1 teaspoon of chopped marjoram or 2 teaspoons of fresh marjoram per cup of water (250ml). You can drink up to 4 cups of this as a digestive after dinner.

For a stronger tea add 2 teaspoons of dried, or 4 teaspoons of fresh, ground leaves to 1 cup of water (250ml) and let sit for 24 hours. Add honey to taste. This stronger marjoram tea is commonly used in Greece and Portugal to aid sleep and relieve mild anxiety.

# MEADOWSWEET

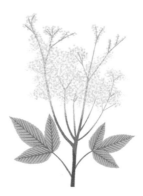

**Other Name** Queen of the meadow.
**Botanical Name** *Filipendula ulmaria.*
**Family** Rosaceae (rose family).
**Parts Used** Leaves, flowers without stems, roots.
**Plant Properties** Pain-relieving, anti-inflammatory, astringent, antiseptic, diaphoretic, diuretic, stomach-soothing.
**Uses** Digestive remedy for heartburn, hyperacidity, nausea, gastritis.
**Preparations** Culinary, pillows, strewing herbs for baths, teas.

**Not suitable for anyone suffering from asthma as it may cause an asthma attack, much like aspirin. Not to be eaten or drunk by pregnant or breastfeeding mothers.**

The smell of meadowsweet on a hot summer's day is so evocative of scrambling out of the streams and rivers of my childhood. It is a wild flower found in damp spots and wet soils, so even when rank growth hides the water's course you can use the meadowsweet to spot where it runs. Meadowsweet is as tall as me, sometimes taller, growing to 1.5 metres in full flower with greyish green, deeply veined leaves and a reddish stem.

Meadowsweet has creamy sprays of tiny flowers that smell of honey, hay and a little of almond with a hint of pine. These flowers have a long history of flavouring drinks, meads, beer and wine, and milky puddings. The leaves have been dried and used to sweeten teas, as well as being widely used as a strewing herb on floors and in pillows due to its fragrance, and it was often known as queen of the meadow. Meadowsweet was used in wedding garlands and strewn across church floors and in houses both to keep the floors warm and to ward off unwanted smells and infections. Apparently this was Queen Elizabeth I's favourite herb for her bedroom and it has been found in the remains of at least three Bronze Age burial chambers, perhaps symbolizing honey-based meads and beers. It is one of the three sacred herbs of the druids (the other two are mint and verbena).

Meadowsweet has an equally long history as a medicinal herb due to its salicylic acid. 'Aspirin' refers to its old botanical name *Spirea ulmaria*. Felix Hoffman, a scientist at Bayer AG, the pharmaceutical company, first created a synthetically altered version of salicin, derived from meadowsweet, in the 1890s. The plant had long been used as a gentle pain reliever and to reduce fevers, but salicin causes less digestive upset than pure salicylic acid, which is one of the reasons why aspirin has gained such widespread use. Meadowsweet roots have tubers that hang off the fibrous root system (it's where '*Filipendula*' comes from – *filium*, meaning thread, and *pendulum*, meaning hanging). These tubers were often chewed for their pain-relieving properties. The tubers were also used with a copper mordant to create black dye.

Much like the drug aspirin, meadowsweet can induce asthma symptoms and the herb should not be used by sufferers for this reason.

# How to grow

Meadowsweet needs to be grown in very damp conditions that most of us don't have. On top of that it grows to be a bit of a beast of a herb, so it's not suitable for small spaces. However, it is widespread through Europe and naturalized in North America, so it's not hard to find it growing locally and forage a little. Two of my local parks have plenty growing and as it's not a herb that you need in huge quantities, sensible small-scale foraging is possible. I tend to use it most as a herb for flavouring seasonal dishes and gather just enough to dry for limited tea use over the winter.

As stated, it needs damp soil, so if you want to grow it, unless you have a stream or river edge, you will need to add a lot of well-rotted compost to the soil to retain moisture. It is best grown in dappled shade or part sun to keep the soil moist. The seed germinates best sown fresh in autumn in rich compost and allowed to sit it out over the winter, where the cold stratification will break the seed's dormancy. When the seedlings are large enough to handle in spring, plant out at least 30cm apart in a well-prepared location. Once established the clumps will need to be divided every three to four years, partly to keep it from overrunning your space and partly to keep the plant vibrant.

# How to use

The very young leaves can be eaten raw or brewed for beer, and they can also be used to sweeten teas. The flowers should be picked when they are just opening, preferably early in the morning and dried on the stem for ease. Once dry it is easy enough to remove flowers from the stems to store.

## Meadowsweet tea

A tea of dried leaves and flowers can be drunk to reduce fevers, muscular pain, colds and flu. Taken very hot it will help sweat out a fever. Meadowsweet tea has a long history of use for treating infant diarrhoea. Cool the tea before giving it to kids. It's very delicious infused in water for 24 hours and drunk with ice.

## For culinary use

I am very fond of meadowsweet-infused rice pudding and custards, where its sweet, subtle perfume and gentle almond-like flavour pervades. It pairs very well with strawberries and so I like to add some when making jam. Strain out the flower heads before bottling. It's delicious sprinkled over fresh fruit salad. You can also make fritters out of the flowers, and unlike elderflower fritters they need no extra sugar. Make a meadowsweet champagne or cordial the same way you might elderflower, but double the quantity of flowers. In fact, meadowsweet can be substituted for elderflower in many recipes, including sorbet.

For those keen on home brewing, experiment with adding meadowsweet for honeyed tones to beers, meads and country wines.

## Meadowsweet rice pudding

I am making no health claims for a pudding that contains over a pint of full-fat milk and plenty of sugar, other than it will lift the spirits and will coax those recovering from an illness into an appetite. It's nursery food for sure. The infused milk part of this recipe can then be used for panna cotta, custards, ice creams and chia teas.

8 heads of meadowsweet with stalks attached

2 pints of full-fat milk or oat milk

200g pudding rice

200g sugar (if you want to reduce your sugar intake, use 100g and try adding two or three stems of sweet cicely. Sweet cicely, as the name suggests, sweetens anything it is added to, but it also adds a hint of aniseed to the flavour.)

Add the meadowsweet heads (and the sweet cicely, if desired) and milk to a saucepan and bring to a rapid boil. Quickly take it off the heat and allow to cool. Steep for at least 15 minutes, but ideally overnight. Strain out the meadowsweet so that you are left with an infused milk. Add the flavoured milk to a heavy-based ovenproof pan with a lid, such as a casserole dish. Add the pudding rice and the sugar, stir briefly, then put in the oven at 180°C/350°F for 40 minutes. The milk may bubble up and over, so stand it on a baking tray to catch any overflow. The top will form a skin and underneath will be perfect clouds of sweet milky rice.

## Meadowsweet vodka

One could make a health claim about alcohol extraction of the plant properties, but let's face it, vodka is going to give you a headache if you drink too much. Still, it's delicious summer fare for sure. It tastes very similar to Żubrówka bison grass vodka.

Eight large heads of meadowsweet, no stalks

1 litre vodka

Fill a quarter of a 1-litre rubber-sealed preserving jar with the flower heads, no stalks, and add the vodka. Leave this to infuse for several days or until the vodka turns a yellow colour. Strain out the flowers and bottle.

## For medicinal use

The root can be chewed for its pain-relieving properties; however, it is illegal to dig up wild-grown plants and it does need a good scrub if you don't want a mouthful of grit. One to park for the zombie apocalypse rather than everyday use. Taking aspirin is a much simpler solution.

# MINT

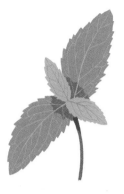

**Other Names** Peppermint, spearmint, horsemint, apple mint, bergamot mint.

**Botanical Names** *Mentha* species.

**Family** Lamiaceae (mint family).

**Parts Used** Entire aerial portion of the plant in flower or not (fresh or dried).

**Plant Properties** Stimulating, cooling, aids digestion, aromatic, carminative, antispasmodic for the digestive tract, mild sedative, local anaesthetic qualities, counterirritant, topical antibacterial agent.

**Uses** For bloating and indigestion, as a temporary decongestant, to relieve tension pains.

**Preparations** Culinary, strewing herb for baths, teas.

Not to be used by people with hiatus hernia. There is some evidence that mint may increase heartburn in some people. The essential oil is incredibly strong and should never be used undiluted, especially on sensitive skin, mucous membranes and eyes. Internal use of the essential oil should only take place under the guidance of a qualified medicinal practitioner.

The coolness of mint, its clean iciness with a hint of black pepper
. . . For all its coolness, once added to water mint tastes fresh,
aromatic and decidedly sweet, only reminding you of its cool after-
taste when you have put the cup down. It has been chewed for as
long as humans have walked, and probably before that too. It thrives
in the dappled damp shade of lakes, rivers and streams, using its long
runners to explore the world around it. Mint is not one to stay still
in the garden; it wanders about finding new territory to colonize,
which is one reason to grow it in a pot.

Mint is a popular and ubiquitous flavour, and can be found in
teas, beverages, jellies, syrups, candies, ice cream and chocolates.
Combined with sugar, mint is heavenly, but it can be utilized in
savoury recipes; paired with parsley in a tabbouleh or with a mild soft
cheese it adds robustness to a salad.

There are around eighteen species of mints, though their taxon-
omy and desire to hybridize readily mean that this number is
contested. Their loose ways with each other result in many hybrids:
ginger mint, *Mentha × gracilis*, which is a cross between field mint, *M.
arvensis*, and spearmint, *M. spicata*, or the equally popular chocolate
mint, *M. × piperita f. citrata* 'Chocolate', which is a cross between
water mint, *M. aquatica*, and spearmint, *M. spicata*.

Everyone has their own favourite mint variety for tea. I personally
think that black-stemmed peppermint, *M. × piperita* 'Black
Peppermint' has a delicious pepperiness to it, but without doubt the
best tea is made from a mixture of mint varieties, which creates a
balance between the heat of the spice and the cool notes. I like
Tashkent mint, *M. spicata* 'Tashkent', with Moroccan mint, *M. spicata*
'Moroccan', and just a hint of apple mint, *M. suaveolens*, which adds
a little fruitiness.

Mint tea is delicious fresh, but the winter may mean slim pickings if you don't force the mint indoors. Therefore it is always worth drying mint for tea. That most kitchen cupboards have teabags of mint tea when it is one of the most simple and easy plants to grow in a pot frankly bothers me. Why do people settle for the stale taste of shop-bought stuff? There's a lot made about picking mint before it flowers for tea, but really you can pick it when you like. The leaves will be a little smaller when it goes into flower, but the flavour of dried flowers adds a new note to the tea, so experiment and see if you like this. Pick dry whole stems and hang them upside down till they crumble. Make sure you dry the mint out of direct sunlight, which will bleach the leaves and reduce the flavour. Store in an airtight container. The stems are full of flavour and can be added to the tea. Avoid over crumbling the tea – just gently break the stems and leaves.

## How to grow

Mint likes dappled shade but can grow equally well in full sun as long as the roots are in rich conditions. It will grow tough in poor soils, which will result in coarse, strongly flavoured leaves that won't be suitable for salads. Add plenty of organic matter if your soil is very free-draining and continue to mulch each year in spring to boost growth. If you are growing mint in a pot (and there is great reason to do this as they can become quite invasive), then you will have to repot every year. As mint spreads through runners or stolons, underground stems that can root, it will quickly grow to the edge of the pot where it will spiral around in a desperate bid to find new ground and the centre of the pot will be bare. Mint left in these conditions grows very poorly, often becoming coarse and bitter. Every spring, just as new growth appears you should tip out the plant from the pot, cut it in half, keeping the section that has the best-looking roots and repot with new compost. This will refresh the plant. Some cut the plant in half and then face the outer edges back to back in the middle of the pot to let the plant grow outwards again. However, I find mint naturally congests the pot and that it's better to start with a small division and let it romp away. The bigger the pot, the more mint you will grow. There is little point in starving a mint in a small pot, so choose one with a 30cm diameter minimum.

If you are desperate for fresh mint in winter and there's none available outside, you can bring a few stolons (the underground stems that are often white) indoors to pot up on your windowsill as a temporary measure. The stolons will quickly start sprouting in the warm conditions.

# How to use

## Mint tea

To make tea use 2 teaspoons of dried crushed leaves or 2 tablespoons of fresh leaves in 1 cup of water (250ml). Cover with a lid or use a teapot to retain the volatile oils and let brew for 10 minutes. Sweeten with honey or sugar if necessary. Most people can drink mint tea all day long and have little issues, but some people are allergic, and react with nausea, headaches and stomach cramps. If you find yourself suffering any of these, stop drinking.

Fresh or dried mint can be infused in water, then left in the sun to brew. Try adding apple, lemon, orange or cucumber to the infusion.

Menthol, the principle chemical in mint, is diaphoretic, meaning it helps you sweat, making mint tea an excellent choice for those with a cold or the flu. Drink mint tea infused for at least 10 minutes, hot or cold, twice a day to help sweat out the infection.

## For medicinal use

Make a poultice with the fresh leaves soaked in hot water and apply to the back, neck or forehead to soothe aches and pains. You can also make a poultice from the dried leaves. Place between layers of muslin or cloth, soak in hot water, and then apply when cool enough to the affected area. There is some folklore that this can alleviate insect bites.

Mint strewn in the bath turns the water a violent green, but it doesn't half make for a lovely refreshing soak. I take mint baths when I have a cold, to revive my respiratory system. Mint's topical antibacterial properties make it a cooling foot bath too. I use big handfuls of fresh mint and sea salt to soak my weary feet as I have a habit of gardening barefoot.

Finally, and it almost goes without saying, chewing mint helps freshen your breath. Chewing mint on its own can be a bit strong, so try adding parsley, which also sweetens your breath, aids digestion and frankly is a much more pleasant experience.

# MYRTLE

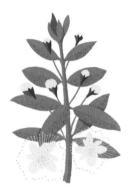

**Botanical Name** *Myrtus communis.*
**Family** Myrtaceae (myrtle family).
**Parts Used** Leaves, berries.
**Plant Properties** Aromatic, antimicrobial, anti-inflammatory, astringent, expectorant, carminative (berries).

**Uses** To relieve dry coughs, sinusitis, to aid digestion and relieve flatulence, gargle for gingivitis.
**Preparations** Culinary, infusions, teas.
**Considerations** May cause asthma in sufferers.

Myrtle is a Mediterranean herb that has been used since antiquity, but is little known outside its sunny, hot baked soils and dry woodlands. It is used widely in southern Italy, Corsica and Sardinia, where the berries or the leaves are used to flavour alcohol with honey to make a drink known as mirto.

Myrtle is packed full of salicylic acid, the precursor to aspirin (see page 182), and has a long folkloric use as a pain reliever, particularly for the respiratory system and painful sinus infections. However, a systematic review of its uses found it had limited benefit.

Myrtle is underused in cooking and is such a pretty evergreen shrub for the garden. Think of it as the glamorous cousin to bay. In summer the whole plant is crowned with sparkling white flowers that are followed late in autumn by dark purple berries. It can be clipped into a hedge or grown in a pot if space is limited. It is quite slow-growing and my small plant has been in a pot for some time, little perturbed by its constricted roots.

## How to grow

Myrtle likes to bake in hot, free-draining soils and needs to be grown somewhere sunny and sheltered. It will not tolerate cold, dry winds. It needs a long hot summer to flower well and fruit will only set in the most sheltered of spots. In much of the UK getting it to fruit is unlikely, but you can grow it in a pot and keep it somewhere sheltered over winter if necessary. It is fairly slow-growing, taking twenty years to reach its ultimate height and width of 2 metres. It is easily clipped to manage its size. It should be pruned mid- to late spring.

## How to use

### For culinary use

Myrtle leaves taste somewhat like bay, with a hint of rosemary and juniper and allspice in there and, like bay, it can be used in soups and stews. It's wonderful with roast meats and can be used with pork, chicken or lamb the way you might rosemary, rubbed or stuffed under the skin. You can also use whole branches of myrtle to flavour meats and fish or in marinades, or to fragrantly smoke meats and fish. The berries can be used in cooking; they have a fruity, slightly astringent flavour. They can be used like you might juniper berries and were once a substitute when dried for pepper, but they are sweet enough to make into a jam if you ever manage to harvest enough.

## For medicinal use

Add a few leaves to hot water for a steam inhalation to relieve sinuses and dry coughs. Cover your head with a towel over the basin for as long as you can bear.

For a mouthwash steep 1 tablespoon of crushed leaves in a cup of boiling water, cool and gargle.

# NETTLE

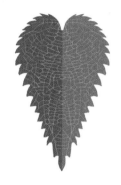

**Other Name**  Stinging nettle.

**Botanical Name**  *Urtica dioicia.*

**Family**  Urticaceae (nettle family).

**Parts Used**  Fresh or dried leaves and stems. The leaves need to be picked when young, ideally before flowers appear.

**Plant Properties**  Astringent, anti-inflammatory, antiseptic, nutritive, diuretic, expectorant.

**Uses**  To reduce hay fever, as a spring tonic, anti-dandruff.

**Preparations**  Culinary, infusions, teas.

**Considerations**  Being stung by one nettle is unpleasant but being stung by lots of nettles is a different thing. I've been kept awake at night almost delirious with the strange buzzing sensation. The antidote is to rub the sting immediately with dock leaves, rosemary or, best of all, with the juice of nettle to dissipate the formic acid. Drinking too much nettle tea can also cause urticaria, which is the term used to describe the red, itchy raised weals you get on the skin. If this happens, stop drinking the tea and drink lots of water. An Epsom salt bath can relieve some of the itching, as will taking an antihistamine tablet.

The nettle is the BDSM of the herb world, those jagged hearts of its leaves hinting at the pain it's about to cause with its needle-like hairs, which are ready to sting at the slightest touch. It's a good defence mechanism to keep munching herbivores away, but stinging nettles have a habit of following humans around. This is partly because human habitation, particularly animal waste (and, before sewers, human waste) increases phosphate and nitrogen in the soil, which nettles love to sup up into their leaves. You can often tell if nettles are growing on poo just from the sheer size of the nettles and the dark green of the leaf. Nitrogen is not good in large doses for our systems. We get rid of phosphate when urinating, but we should still be wary of eating or drinking too much of this herb, particularly if you've found it growing on recent manure. Nettles don't tend to grow on fresh manure, but even a year-old pile will be rich in nitrogen. Too much of either element is toxic to our systems.

Nettles can be rotted down to make an excellent compost tea to feed your plants. You can either rot the nettles down in water until it's the colour of weak tea, or you can add them to comfrey for a more rounded nutritious feed. Or, if you find yourself with a magnificent pile of nettles to harvest, steal a trick from biodynamic growers and make a nettle soil. This can be made by digging a hole in the ground, lining the sides with wood, then packing in the nettles as tightly as possible. Then cover with a stone or bit of wood and leave for several months. The nettles will rot down into the softest black compost imaginable. This is the stuff to start seedlings off in, sprinkle a little down seed drills in the garden, or mix in with compost to start seeds off in pots. You can also use thinly to top-dress perennial plants in pots, where it will act as both a feed and a mulch.

We've been crypto-cropping nettles for as long as we can remember. Crypto-crop is a strange ethnobotanical term to describe a method of semi-cultivating a wild crop to harvest. We allow certain weeds to grow in the margins of our fields and provide just enough love to make sure they are always abundant. Nettles have a long history as a food source, medicine and raw material for textiles. Vikings used nettle fibres to weave with, and both the roots and leaves can be used as a dye. The roots produce a deep yellow and the leaves a yellow-green colour.

The spring harvest of nettles is still widespread; from Italy to America you can find people plucking the tips for pasta, risottos, soups, smoothies or just as greens. You can also eat the young stolons, which boil up rather nicely. The young leaves should be cooked very briefly – no more than 60 seconds to keep both their fresh green colour and their nutritional content. The leaves contain appreciable amounts of protein, fatty acids, omega-3s, vitamins A and C, iron, potassium, manganese and calcium. In peak season nettle leaves can contain up to 25 per cent protein by dry weight, which is very high for a leafy green. These leaves truly are a spring tonic after a winter of limited greens.

Nettles can be used in brewing for nettle beer; young shoots are used for this process.

## How to grow

Ha! You truly do not have to grow nettles; they will come to your garden of their own accord. The best nettles can be found in fertile, rich ground in dappled shade. However, you should abide by a few foraging lores. Always wear gloves, otherwise you will spend all night feverish with itchy hands red with welts. Pick in spring before the flowers appear, because once the flowers appear the leaves develop gritty particles known as cystoliths, which can act as an irritant to the kidneys and digestive system.

# How to harvest

The fresh leaves and young shoots should be picked from early to late spring. Mechanical damage or boiling water will kill the stings, making them safe to eat. The nettle leaves are very pleasant to eat raw; roll over them with a rolling pin several times to break the glass-like structure of the sting. Submerging the leaves in boiling water or heat will also subdue the sting. Nettles should only very briefly be cooked; if you want to make a soup, create a broth and add the nettles at the very end of cooking. They certainly shouldn't be boiled.

## To dry

Cut whole stems from May to June before flowering and hang upside down somewhere with good air circulation, but out of the sun. Once paper-dry store in an airtight container.

The roots can be harvested at any point in the year, and scrubbed and dried for use as a dye.

# How to use

## Nettle tea

Nettles have been recognized for their anti-inflammatory properties, particularly for allergens. Nettle tea is the simplest way to take this herb medicinally for daily use. The tea tastes a little bland, so you can add other ingredients to improve the flavour. Traditionally elder-flower and plantain, with their antiviral and immune-stimulating properties, are a good seasonal addition to fresh leaves. I like the fruity flavour of blackcurrant leaves. Similarly you can infuse nettle water for 24 hours with cucumber, lemon and cleavers to make a spring tonic to boost your immune system. After that time you will start to notice the water and herbs begin to ferment, so it's best to make small batches regularly, rather than large quantities.

For tea use 1–2 teaspoons of dried nettle or 1–2 tablespoons of fresh nettle per cup of water (250ml), steeped with a lid or in a teapot for 10 minutes. You can drink up to 3 cups a day to fight hay fever, as well as the symptoms of other environmental pollutants.

## Apple cider vinegar and nettle hair tonic

Nettles also make an excellent hair tonic; a decoction of the seeds is said to help stimulate hair growth and the dried herb improves the texture and tone of the hair. Its antiseptic, anti-inflammatory proper-ties also help against dandruff. This tonic should be used after shampooing and conditioning. Cider vinegar also promotes a healthy scalp and makes your hair shine. Rosemary is added for the same reasons, but also to make the mixture smell nice and it also slightly darkens the hair. If you don't want the darkening effect of rosemary, use a few drops of rosemary oil rather than the fresh herb. If you have light hair, you could substitute camomile for rosemary.

5 tablespoons dried nettle or 15 tablespoons fresh nettle (aka a big bunch, stalks included)

1 large sprig of rosemary (optional)
400ml water
100ml apple cider vinegar

Add the nettles and rosemary to the water, bring to the boil and simmer for 20 minutes. The water should be the colour of dark tea. Allow the mixture to cool and strain off the liquid, then add the cider vinegar. Store in a spray bottle and keep in the fridge to prevent the mixture from fermenting. This mixture will keep for at least a month.

Some people prefer to rinse this tonic through the hair. After shampooing leave the tonic on for at least 3 minutes before rinsing out. It's perfectly acceptable to leave it on if you like, though your hair will smell of rosemary and vinegar. Concentrate the liquid on the scalp and roots, brush your hair afterwards and style as normal. If you wash your hair daily, you may want to reduce the vinegar content and just use 50ml of cider vinegar.

# OATS

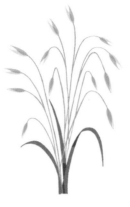

**Other Names** Common oats, wild oats, common wild oats, sterile oats.

**Botanical Names** *Avena sativa, Avena barbata, Avena fatua, Avena sterilis.*

**Family Name** Poaceae (grass family).

**Parts Used** Young 'milky' oats, all aerial parts when young and green collected for oat straw.

**Plant Properties** Nervine, diuretic, nutritive.

**Uses** To treat exhaustion, sleeplessness and stress.

**Preparations** Baths, culinary, teas.

**Considerations** Oats contain avenin, a similar protein to gluten, and may cause sensitivity in those with a gluten intolerance.

I am a huge fan of oat straw tea, particularly at bedtime. I use oat straw, which is the green parts of the oat plant, but not the oats, in conjunction with any number of other herbs to make a restful night-time brew. You'll often find oat straw in commercial sleep and night-time teas. It is said to treat exhaustion, sleeplessness and restlessness. It also tastes lovely, grass-like with a sweetness that rounds off the tea pleasantly.

I grow two types of cultivated oats, one that came as a volunteer via the birds from a wild birdseed mixture and the other a naked oat. 'Naked' means that the oat is hull-less and needs little processing to create groats, the unrolled oats that can be cooked like rice or into porridge. They are delicious, highly nutritious and a very easy-to-grow cereal for small-scale home production. I grow the oats in clumps throughout the garden, like you might ornamental grasses. They are a very pleasing pale green and sway delightfully in the wind.

The wild oats, the slender wild oat, *Avena barbata*, the common wild oat, *A. fatua*, and the wild or sterile oat, *A. sterilis*, can all be used interchangeably with the cultivated form for medicinal purposes.

I harvest the wild birdseed oat for milk oats and the oat straw for tea. Milk oats are immature seeds that when pressed release a white milky substance. They must be harvested the minute the milky sap appears as it's a small window before they mature and dry. If you cut the oat to just above ground level, you'll often get a second flush of green leaves and stems that can be harvested in late summer. I tend to harvest both the straw and the milky oats at the same time, hanging them up to dry and then running my hand along the oat seeds to release them. I chop up the oat straw when it's perfectly dry. You can use both the milky oats and the oat straw interchangeably in tea.

The naked oats I leave until they ripen on the plant in late summer, when the whole thing has turned straw-coloured. These I thrash by gently hitting the plant on a clean sheet, which is usually all that is needed to remove the seed. You can then remove any chaff by winnowing. One of the simplest ways to winnow is to use a fan somewhere you don't mind the chaff blowing about and gently toss the oats in a wide flat bowl in front of the fan. The chaff will blow out of the bowl, probably all over you if you stand in front rather than to the side of the fan, and the seed, being heavier, will drop back in.

# How to grow

Oats are annuals. In the UK, you can sow them in autumn and again in spring. They take roughly fifty days to harvest for milky oat tops after a spring sowing. Oats like well-drained fertile soil in full sun. The plants are tall and may need support if not grown in a dense block. Sow the seed direct, covering with mesh, otherwise the pigeons and squirrels will have them, or sow in modules, planting out when the green tops have two leaves and an established root system. Plant the modules very close together, 1–2cm apart, as the oats seem to benefit from neighbourly support. Unharvested, oats will self-seed everywhere.

# How to use

## Oat tea

Milky oats, fresh or dried, or oat straw can be made into a tea. Use 1–2 teaspoons of dried material or 1–2 tablespoons of fresh in 1 cup of boiling water, covering to steep for 10 minutes. You can drink up to 4 cups a day. It's a very calming tea and won't send you to sleep per se, so you can drink this throughout the day if you wish.

## Oat straw for baths

Oat straw is great for reducing irritation and inflammation and can temporarily relieve itching. Tie two or three large handfuls in a muslin bag to soften the water and skin, or add to the warm bath and soak for 20 minutes. You can also add rolled porridge oats to this recipe if you want to make it slightly stronger.

# OREGANO,
## *see* MARJORAM

---

# PARSLEY

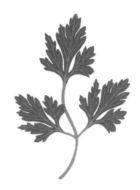

**Other Name**  Garden parsley.

**Botanical Name**  *Petroselinum crispum.*

**Family**  Apiaceae (carrot family).

**Parts Used**  Fresh leaves, stems and roots.

**Plant Properties**  Digestion, nutritive, carminative, diuretic.

**Uses**  To relieve bloating and bad breath, anti-dandruff.

**Preparations**  Culinary, poultices, teas.

**Considerations**  Large doses of parsley are not suitable for pregnant women as there is some suggestion that it may weaken the uterus and induce early labour.

Parsley is my desert island herb; it's the one I'd run into the waves to save. Basil is fruity, a little flirty even, mint may be cool, thyme has its spice and rosemary its sweet smell, but parsley with dark green glossy leaves is the green I most often crave. To me a good salad always has at least a big handful of parsley. I love its clean, earthy taste. I think once you begin eating parsley regularly, you truly get addicted to its fix. And there is plenty of reason to eat lots of fresh parsley. It's rich in polyphenols, flavonoids and other antioxidants, especially luteolin and apigenin, the latter of which has been found in some studies to play a role in adult neurogenesis (the process by which neurons are generated), which reportedly plays a role in learning, memory, emotions, stress, depression and response to injury. The jury is still out, but I for one am very happy to eat lots of parsley if it helps to make my brain function just a tiny bit better.

On top of all of the antioxidants in fresh parsley it also contains appreciable amounts of folic acid and vitamins A, C and K. Vitamins K and A are fat-soluble and your body absorbs them best if you eat them with a source of fat. Parsley and olive oil are a marriage made in gut heaven. Vitamin K is particularly good for your blood and is important in bone health and, much like kales and other leafy greens, it's packed with the stuff, particularly K1. Vitamin K is a group made up of vitamin K1 and K2. K1 is a phylloquinone and is made by plants, particularly leafy greens. Animals, including us, convert K1 into K2. Our bodies can store K2 for longer. Thirty grams of raw parsley has over 500 per cent of the recommended daily amount of K1, and unlike kale it's much easier to eat raw, as cooking destroys much of the vitamin K. It is also an excellent source of folate, which helps to keep homocysteine levels low. High levels of homocysteine are linked to heart disease.

Parsley is native to the Mediterranean but is widely naturalized across Europe. It is a biennial or short-lived perennial, and once it flowers and sets seed it gives up the ghost. The flowers are small, white and rather pretty. They are much loved by the bees and pollinators and the seed is particularly appealing to finches over winter, so it's well worth letting it flower if you have the space in your garden.

Parsley doesn't have a particularly extensive history medicinally and is often overlooked, but it does seem to aid digestion, reduce flatulence and is a good diuretic. There's quite a lot of folkloric use for parsley tea, particularly the roots, to reduce oedema and swelling, particularly swollen ankles.

# How to grow

Parsley seed is notoriously slow to germinate, taking up to six weeks if the seed is a little old. This is because the seed coat is covered in furanocoumarins, which are toxic to animals and are there to prevent insects and mammals from eating them. Parsley doesn't have the most toxic furanocoumarins (those are in giant hogweed and wild parsnips, which can cause skin blistering if the sap is exposed to sunlight), but you shouldn't chow down on the seed. I find the trick is to make sure that the seed germinates around 22–30°C/70–86°F, so sow indoors in spring, and ensure that the soil is not allowed to dry out until germination occurs. Parsley is fairly drought-tolerant once it is allowed to get its roots down, but they do need space. It has an extensive root system, at least 30–50cm deep, and growing parsley in a tiny pot will make it weedy, weak and turn brown in full sun.

# How to use

### For culinary use
Parsley tea may have its history, but frankly it doesn't taste good and a much simpler way to enjoy parsley is to eat it.

Tabbouleh should be stuffed with parsley, overflowing with it, and then a little mint. Use a ratio of five parts parsley to one part mint, a good fresh tomato or two, and just a small amount of cracked wheat or freekeh, all dressed with plenty of lemon juice, good oil and a smattering of smashed garlic and a good pinch of salt. This is the simplest and most enjoyable way to eat a bunch of parsley.

But parsley should not be resigned to tabbouleh alone. Year-round it is a great salad ingredient, which works wonderfully in salsa verdes and German green sauces, mixed with lemon balm, salad burnet and chives. It is also the best ingredient for potatoes; mint is fine for new ones, but all the others, better still a good floury main crop, should be drenched in parsley whether they've been roasted, or boiled to perfection with that outer layer just starting to flake away . . . With the gentle pressing of the back of the fork they crumble, hopefully into a pool of butter dotted liberally with good parsley.

Then, of course, there is a good gremolata, woefully underused, but the perfect way to get your dose of garlic and parsley and lemon. Add the juice and zest of a lemon to a large bunch of parsley, stems and leaves minced, and a clove or two or three of crushed garlic and some good flaky salt. This can be used to dress fish or swirled over pasta dripping in oil. Alternatively it can be added as a last-minute seasoning to osso buco and is so good I sometimes just make it as a salad and eat it alone. You can make a very pungent version using preserved lemon rind if you're after a salt kick. If you forgo the lemon and use olive oil, you have a rudimentary salsa verde or chimichurri, which is excellent for meat or dipping good sourdough bread into.

Finally you can make a pesto of parsley using the usual suspects: pine nuts, walnuts or hazelnuts, parmesan (or you could use Emmental or

Gouda instead), olive oil, garlic and then lemon juice. You could also add a little coriander, some other greens, such as bitter dandelion leaves or lemon balm, salad burnet, even plantain leaves. At this point I'm not sure you could still call it a pesto, but this sauce is great for pasta or spread on meats, for dipping into or, better still, with scrambled eggs for breakfast.

# PERILLA

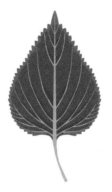

**Other Names** Shiso, Korean perilla, Japanese basil.

**Botanical Name** *Perilla frutescens*.

**Family** Lamiaceae (mint family).

**Parts Used** Leaves, seeds.

**Plant Properties** Anti-inflammatory, nutritive, antibacterial, expectorant, wound-healing.

**Uses** For coughs and colds, cuts and abrasions.

**Preparations** Culinary, infusions, teas.

**Considerations** None known.

*Perilla frutescens* is an annual native to South East Asia where it is widely used in cooking. Most will know it, if not by sight, by taste from Japanese food, where it often features both as a vegetable and to flavour and colour other foods. The deep red version of *P. frutescens* 'Crispa', with its curly leaves, is used to colour pickled ume plums a violent violet and, sometimes, to turn pickled ginger an equally vibrant shade. The green form is often paired with glutinous rice and shredded in salads. It is also widely used in Korean food where it is pickled either as a kangajii or as a kimchi and can be used fresh as a vegetable. In China both the seed and leaves are widely combined with red bean paste to make a bun. In India the seeds are eaten raw and can be roasted and ground to make a spicy chutney, and the seed oil is used in cooking. In the UK until recently we mainly used it as a bedding plant for Victorian park schemes. It's a very pretty-looking thing, but what a waste to just look at it when there's eating to be had.

In north-eastern Japan, perilla is known *jūnen*, which translates as 'ten years', and this is supposedly because it adds many years to your lifespan. It is certainly full of dietary minerals, vitamins and fibre, such as vitamins A and C and riboflavin. And there is much work underway looking into the oil from the seed, which is so rich in Omega-3 fatty acids that it has been linked to the prevention of diseases such as cardiovascular disorders and inflammatory and rheumatoid arthritis. It has traditionally been used for its anti-inflammatory properties. Perilla is used in Chinese medicine for digestive ailments as it has antibacterial and anti-inflammatory benefits. It may play some role in reducing allergy symptoms when eaten regularly. A tea made from the leaves is used in Chinese medicine to treat coughs and cold symptoms. The juice of the leaves can be used on minor cuts and abrasions because of its antibacterial properties.

## How to grow

There are two variants of *P. frutescens* to grow: the green types, which are most widely used for cooking (sometimes this type has a red underside to the leaves), and the dark metallic red *P. frutescens* 'Crispa', which is used mostly for pickling and dyeing.

The seed needs to be fresh to germinate quickly and it is not always easy to get hold of good stock. However, I've found that soaking the seed for four to eight hours before sowing can speed things up. Once you have rinsed the seed from soaking, treat it just like you would basil. Grow it somewhere warm, germinating at around 20°C/68°F and prick on, keeping it indoors until all threat of frost has passed. It is manna to slugs when young, but tough when older, so bear that in mind; it can be grown in the ground, but it seems to thrive best in pots in sunny corners. It's highly attractive, but, in truth, unless you are using the seed you don't need many plants.

# How to use

### For culinary use
Experiment with using it in your cooking. I like to shred the younger leaves into rice or use it to wrap other foods. It works well with fish and I often add it to polenta too. It can make the base of an Asian-style salad when dressed with fish sauce and rice wine vinegar.

My favourite use of the plant is to take a handful of leaves, say six or seven, and steep them in 350ml of cider, white wine or rice vinegar for a month. If you use the purple perilla, then the mixture will go a wonderful deep red. The vinegar tastes decidedly fruity and it's one way to capture some of the benefits of perilla deep into winter when the plant is long gone.

# PINES

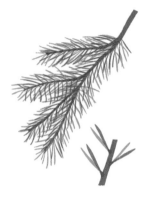

**Botanical Names** *Pinus* species.
**Family** Pinaceae (pine family).
**Parts Used** Pine needles.
**Plant Properties** Antimicrobial, decongestant, improves circulation.
**Uses** Coughs, colds, congestion, muscle aches and pains.

**Preparations** Strewing herb for baths.
**Considerations** Some people are very sensitive to the Pinaceae family and therefore should avoid this plant.

I am not expecting you to grow a pine tree in your herb garden, but these are useful trees both in culinary and medicinal terms. The Scots pine is our native and most prominent member of the pine family, found everywhere from car parks to seaside woodlands and, of course, all over Scotland. Pine needles are deeply aromatic with a clean, fresh scent that comes from its essential oils, pinenes. These essential oils are well-known decongestants and are antimicrobial, so they can be used in steam baths or in the tub to help open up airways that have been closed by coughs, colds and respiratory issues. You can also infuse the needles in oils, such as olive, jojoba or almond, and then massage into the skin to help ease muscle ache. It is also possible to make a tea from the very young needles; this has a powerful pine taste, but is very rich in vitamin C.

## How to forage

*Be very careful not to mistake a yew tree for pines.* Poisoning from a yew tree will induce vomiting, abdominal pain, drowsiness, dizziness, coma and, in extreme cases, death. The needles of yews are short and arranged like a double-sided comb. The needle ends are hard and pointed, dark green above and yellowish-green below. Yew trees are the only conifer that produces true berries, which are pinkish red and shaped like a cup with a brown seed clearly visible inside.

## How to use

The eastern white pine, *Pinus strobus*, makes an excellent and very delicious tea, if you can find it; the young tips are also edible and fairly sweet. The white pine can be identified by its bundles of five needles that are flexible, bluish-green and finely serrated. This tree is native to northern America, so you will most likely find it in parks and amenity plantings.

Finally the Norway Spruce, *Picea abies*, which is a tall conifer, growing up to 60 metres high, with reddish-brown bark and is distinctly Christmas tree-shaped when young. Its needles are 10–25mm long, four-sided and end in a very sharp point. The cones hang down from the branches and are 9–17cm long. This is a common Christmas tree and the young needles make a delicious syrup. The young shoots harvested in mid-spring are edible and can be added to breads, used in marinades, desserts (pine ice cream is really something) or infused in olive oil for cooking with. The young male cones can also be infused in olive oil for the same purpose. The spring needles are very rich in vitamin C and can also be made into a tea to drink.

When making tea from any of these trees make sure you don't boil the needles as vitamin C is very heat-sensitive and is quickly destroyed in such conditions. Boil the water, then pour it over the needles and infuse for 10 minutes before drinking.

# PLANTAIN

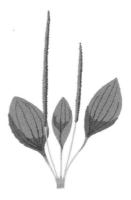

**Other Names** Ribwort or narrow-leaved plantain, broadleaf plantain, hoary plantain.

**Botanical Names** *Plantago lanceolata* (ribwort plantain), *Plantago major* (broadleaf plantain), *Plantago media* (hoary plantain).

**Family** Plantaginaceae (plantain family).

**Parts Used** Leaves and stems (fresh or dried). Seeds when mature.

**Plant Properties** Antiseptic, astringent, antimicrobial, anti-inflammatory, antihistamine, demulcent, expectorant, styptic, diuretic.

**Uses** Spring tonic, skin problems, minor wounds, drawing poultice.

**Preparations** Compresses, culinary, poultices, teas.

**Considerations** None known.

You might not have noticed plantains in the UK. Those in the know may have seen them only as the weeds of waysides, paths and very neglected lawns. Or perhaps you are thinking of the banana relative? *Plantago* is a genus of about 200 species found all over the world. The name *plantago* refers in Latin to the sole of a foot, the suffix -ago meaning 'a sort of'. One might like to think this somehow refers to the fact that plantains are very good at drawing out splinters and infections, but no, it refers to the fact that many of these species, particularly the broadleaf plantain, when grown in poor conditions grow near flat at ground level. In short, it refers to the fact that you have probably walked on this plant.

All plantains are characterized by thick, mid-green leaves in a rosette with very prominent ribs that run along the entire leaf. A trick when identifying the plant is to pull the leaf away from the ribs, which will remain intact, like string. The flowers of the ribwort plantain, *P. lanceolata*, appear at the end of tall stems in a rounded, club-like spike of tiny brownish-green flowers surrounded by a corona of stamens. The leaves are long, narrow and deep green. The broadleaf, *P. major*, has flat, spade-like leaves with a short stem and the flowers appear on a long green spike that resembles a rat's tail – its other common name. *P. media*, the hoary plantain, sits between the two species, though the basal rosette of leaves is very flat to the ground and it has delicate pink-white flowers between May and September.

Plantain leaves in a tea is very good for tickly coughs and sore throats. It should be mixed with something like marjoram, lemon balm, lemon verbena or mint, as the astringent nature of the leaves can be a little mouth-puckering. It can be added to nettle tea where its demulcent and anti-inflammatory properties will aid with hay fever. The mashed-up leaves make an excellent drawing poultice, which has been used since prehistoric times as a herbal remedy for extracting the unwanted from the skin. These poultices can be used to draw out insect bites, poison ivy, rashes, minor sores, boils, acne and eczema, as well as for toothache and abscesses. It is the go-to herb to use under a plaster.

The species *P. psyllium*, which is native to the Mediterranean, is used commercially for its seed husks, which expand and become mucilaginous when wet, and are a common bulk laxative and fibre in many commercial supplement products. The seed is edible and often considered a good survival food as it is rich in fatty acids. The alpine plantain, *P. alpina*, has large seeds that are certainly worth snacking on if you find some on a long mountain walk. The alpine variety is also the prettiest of all plantain in my opinion, with its soft, baby pink flowers that fade to cotton white, though it's almost impossible to buy as a plant, so you have to collect seeds yourself.

## How to grow

Both ribwort and broad-leaved plantains are native weeds to the UK, so you can forage easily once you know to look in damp, fertile, semi-shaded spots of longer grass and the margins of grassland, fields and hedge edges. However, it is possible to either collect ripe seed from foraged plants or buy from a reputable wildflower seed merchant and grow your own crop. I think this method is preferable because the best plants are grown in fertile, moisture-rich ground and you can be sure they are free from any contaminants, such as dog pee or, worse still, herbicides.

# How to use

## Plantain tea

For tea add 1–2 teaspoons of dried herb to 250ml of boiled water and infuse for 10 minutes. Or add 1–2 tablespoons of fresh herb.

## For culinary use

The broadleaf plantain, *P. major*, is a highly nutritious leaf vegetable, rich in calcium and vitamins A, C and K. Only the younger leaves are palatable; the older ones are just too tough and astringent. There is also a staghorn or buck's horn plantain, *P. coronopus*, which has slightly succulent leaves and a nutty flavour. You often find it eaten in Italy where it is called *erba stella* or *minutina*. It's very pretty and a nice addition to the salad garden and herbal tea if you can find the seed.

## For medicinal use

The fresh mashed-up or bruised leaves of any plantain species can be used in a poultice that should be changed regularly, every couple of hours if necessary.

To make a drawing poultice for a swollen gum or tooth, mash up the leaves and place in a layer of clean cheesecloth, shaping into a small bolus (a small ball-like shape). This can then be placed between the gum and the lip of the swollen gum or tooth.

For insect stings and bites, work the leaves between your hands until moist as this breaks open the cell structures and releases the chemical constituents. Rub on the affected part as often as needed. Plantain will act as a natural antibacterial and antihistamine.

# POPPIES

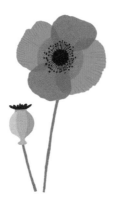

**Botanical Names** *Eschscholzia california* (Californian poppy), *Papaver rhoeas* (field poppy).

**Family** Papaveraceae (poppy family).

**Parts Used** Flowers, leaves, seed heads, seeds.

**Plant Properties** Sedative, analgesic, diaphoretic, antispasmodic.

**Uses** Insomnia, anxiety, headaches, tension.

**Preparations** Culinary, teas.

**Considerations** Although it is considered safe for children, it should not be used for infants. It is recommended to speak to a medical practitioner before using for children.

**Not to be used in pregnancy.**

I grew up in a house that felt the need to remind us not to become opium addicts every time we went to the loo. The illustrations to Thomas De Quincey's *Confessions of an English Opium-Eater* hung in the bathroom and the last part where opium sucks the life out of ravaged de Quincey's body while the opium poppies flower voluptuously from human skulls was a daily reminder to not chase the dragon, as my father put it. This was at slight odds with the fact that he taught us all how to score the opium poppies to release the sticky latex that is turned into the drug opium.

Poppies contain twenty-five different alkaloids, but none of the others have quite the same effects as the opiates on our bodies. They are a powerful pain relief, but an addictive one. We've been extracting opium from poppies for its numbing, nulling opiate haze and abusing these properties for as long as they have been used for our benefit too.

Many old herbals provide recipes for opium tea, which is usually made from the dried poppy seed heads. Every day millions of people consume the same poppies for their seeds. I can tell you plenty on how to grow opium poppies for bread seed but legally I am not allowed to tell you how to make a 'warm bath' or a tea for backache. Perhaps rightly so.

What I can tell you about is the laid-back West Coast alternative, the Californian poppy, *Eschscholzia californica* or our own humble field poppy, *Papaver rhoeas*, both of which have just as long a history as their potent cousin for pain relief, sedative properties and easing anxiety. As the alkaloids present in these poppies are mild and gentle they can be used to promote a deep and dreamless sleep.

## How to grow

Both the Californian poppy and the field poppy are cheerful annuals. If you are lucky enough to have a mild winter, the former can be a short-lived perennial. They like to waft about in the short, sparse grasses of scrublands and meadows, and before big agriculture took over our fields, *P. rhoeas* would grow in our wheat, barley and cereal crops. They both have showy, simple cup-shaped flowers, though the California poppy is brilliant orange and sometimes yellow, with a glaucous grey-green foliage and a long, thin seed head. The field poppy is usually brilliant-red with a black centre, but can equally come in every shade from red to palest pink and almost white and yellow. The field poppies' delicate blooms last a single day, but in a warm and not too dry season, a single plant can produce up to 400 flowers. Its seed heads are cup-shaped capsules.

Like most poppies, both plants do best in disturbed soil with little competition. They should be sown in full sun, in soil that is free from weeds and other plants. The seeds are often tiny and light sensitive, meaning it will fail to germinate if shaded out from other plants. It should be surface-sown for this reason too. Sow in autumn for early-summer flowering or from around March for summer flowering. Early-autumn sowing often produces a better crop, particularly for the field poppy. Once you have established both plants in your garden or pots, then it is possible to just allow them to self-seed, remembering that if your space becomes too overcrowded with other plants then you may lose them. These plants do best by being allowed to move around as they please, often favouring path edges, shingle and gravelly spaces, so remember to leave some seed for this purpose.

## How to use

Collect leaves, flowers and seedpods – the latter need to be collected before the seedpods split open. All parts can be used fresh or dried.

## Poppy tea

Make a basic tea using 1–2 teaspoons of dried herb to 250ml of boiling water and allow it to infuse for 10 minutes. Drink a single cup of tea before bed to aid sleep. This tea can be combined with camomile or lime blossom to make a pleasing bedtime tea.

## For culinary use

The seeds are edible and can be added to bread. Alternatively mix them with honey in equal parts to make a paste. This can be dissolved into tea or taken on its own before bedtime or to help with a tickly cough. The seed is easily stored in an airtight container and it's best to make this paste up as needed.

# RASPBERRY

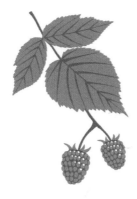

**Botanical Name** *Rubus idaeus.*
**Family** Rosacea (rose family).
**Parts Used** Leaves, berries.
**Plant Properties** Astringent, anti-inflammatory, birthing aid.
**Uses** Strengthens and tones the uterus before going into labour. Also used to ease diarrhoea, and as a mouthwash and gargle for sore throats.
**Preparations** Culinary, infusions, teas.
**Considerations** Raspberry leaf can cause uterine contractions and should therefore be avoided in early pregnancy.

Raspberry leaf has such a long tradition of use in pregnancy to help strengthen and tone the uterus that it is one of those herbs that many people know about, particularly if they have children, when it is usually used in the last trimester as a uterine tonic and toner. Raspberry leaf tea has no side effects or known drug interactions and can be drunk freely, either as a hot tea or infused into water. Raspberry leaves are pleasant but don't exactly have a pronounced flavour, so when infusing the water, try adding other ingredients, such as raspberries themselves, pomegranate seeds, nettles, goji berries or lemon in any number of combinations. Its natural astringent properties mean that raspberry leaf tea is good for sore throats and mouth ulcers and makes a good general tonic.

Raspberries grow wild over great tracts of the world and if you can find a good, clean, unpolluted spot I do think wild raspberries are a lovely thing to forage for. You should pick the leaf in late spring/early summer before the flowers appear when it's most green and vibrant-looking. The taste of wild raspberries is really something, but they disintegrate as you pick them so they are for nibbling on the job rather than collecting. However, you can make a fine raspberry vodka in a good wild raspberry year and although any health benefits will be drastically reduced by the alcohol, the joy of the flavour (in moderation, of course) must have some positive effect on one's overall well-being.

You can dry the leaves very easily by placing them on a clean tea towel or pillowcase and leaving them somewhere airy and dry. If you have a rambunctious patch of raspberries, you might consider cutting and drying whole branches for ease, though it's mainly the younger upper leaves that you're after.

## How to grow

Raspberries love to run about the place; they are hard to keep in a permanent spot and want to roam about via their extensive underground roots that travel not that far below the surface of the soil. At woodland edges raspberries grow in shallow leaf litter and move about to search for minerals and nutrients. They are a hungry lot and their runners allow them to head off in the direction they perceive to be fullest of food. Despite their nomadic nature, we see fit to treat them otherwise and insist that they sit in the same spot, often grown in a straight line, tethered to a wire support. Raspberries resent this and send up endless suckers under the garden path through the fruit cage in the direction they would prefer to move. If you have the space (and raspberries really won't like pots for more than a year or two), let them roam and worry little about feeding them. If you don't have such space and must keep them happy in the same spot, then mulch them in spring and autumn with well-rotted material, dried comfrey leaves, leaf mould or garden- or shop-bought compost. If you don't do this, you'll find that the leaves start to show nutrient deficiencies in early summer, often prematurely turning pale yellow or mottling with greener veins to the leaves, as a healthy plant usually would in late summer, when the leaves naturally start to decline after fruiting.

There are two types of cultivated raspberries, summer- and autumn-fruited types, and these need to be pruned differently to ensure a fruiting crop. Summer raspberries fruit on second-year canes, the previous year's growth, and these are pruned out after fruiting. This is very apparent as you'll have lots of new healthy, vibrant green canes appearing and the older ones with spent fruit stalks will start to go yellow. Prune these out around the end of July/August. Autumn raspberries fruit on this year's cane, that's the current season's growth, and they should be chopped down in early spring around February. Cut every cane back to ground level. If you have no idea whether your raspberry is autumn- or summer-fruiting, cut everything back in February. Then, if you don't get any fruit in the autumn, you'll know that you have summer-fruiting canes, which will fruit the following year. Clearly pruning is not necessary for raspberry leaf, but however healthy this tea is, raspberry plants are mostly worth growing for those lovely berries.

# How to use

## Raspberry tea

Pour 1 cup (250ml) of boiling water over 2 teaspoons of dried herbs or 2 tablespoons of fresh leaves, then cover and infuse for 10–15 minutes.

If you are making an infusion, the leaves need to soak for a minimum of 4 hours, but are best after 12–24 hours in the fridge.

Both drinks may be drunk freely as there are no known side effects.

# Other species

Blackberry, *Rubus fructicosus*, is a very safe astringent. The berries, leaves and very young shoots can all be used for their gentle toning properties against diarrhoea and dysentery or other issues with loose bowels. You can also use a wash of berries and leaves to treat minor burns and skin irruptions. The crushed berries will act as a styptic to stem bleeding and aid scab formation. The young blackberry leaves can be used as a tea, much like raspberry, to strengthen the uterus and relieve heavy periods.

# ROSE

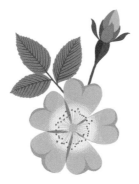

**Botanical Name** *Rosa* species.

**Family** Rosaceae (rose family).

**Parts Used** Hips, flowers, the very youngest leaves.

**Plant Properties** Astringent, anti-inflammatory, diuretic, sedative.

**Uses** Colds, flu, sore throats, diarrhoea, skin health, anxiety.

**Preparations** Culinary, strewing herb for baths, teas.

**Considerations** The seeds of rose hips are covered in hairs that will irritate the stomach and need to be removed if you are processing the hips for jam or sauces.

Not all roses are born equal and, although in theory any rose petal is edible, many are overbred. The thick, waxy petals of a double show rose are a far cry from the soft, delicate flavour of a wild dog rose, *Rosa canina*, or for that matter from the heavenly scent of *R. × damascena*, which is used worldwide in cosmetic and beauty products. The properties of many bred roses for medicinal and healthful purposes are not widely known and, as in all of these things, those that are closest to their wild ancestor probably have more potency. The thicker, fleshier leaves of bred roses are also hard to cook with as they toughen rapidly, so in all cases go for simple open-cup-shaped flowers with smaller petals. Roses are gentle and effective astringents; the flowers, flower buds and young leaves can be used for toning and for inflamed skin complaints; from sore throats to mild diarrhoea or acne, rose water or a rosebud infusion is a pleasant solution.

Dry the petals and grind them into a powder, then mix with equal parts honey to take when your stomach is upset or your throat sore.

Rose hips are a powerful source of vitamin C, antioxidants and flavonoids, which are anti-inflammatory. Vitamin C is rather rapidly destroyed when boiled for too long, so if you are making a rosehip syrup, bear this in mind. The hairs inside the hips are an irritant to the stomach lining and skin and so need to be removed before processing. Some suggest drying hips first and then breaking them up in a blender so that the hairs can be sieved out, but I find this very messy and prefer to choose fat hips, which I split and scoop out when fresh and then dry. I find if you split the hips in a bowl of water the hairs are far less irritating.

The real trick, though, is to go for *R. rugosa*, the tomato or beach rose that is not native to this part of the world, but so widely planted and naturalized that it is easy enough to find in inner cities or at the seaside. The flowers are large, pink or white, and the whole plant is often grown as a loose informal hedge. It is a trouble-free sort, little bothered by normal rose diseases and therefore is often used in municipal plantings and alongside roads where it is unfazed by de-icing salt. After the bright pink flowers come fat hips, which are bright tomato orange, hence its name. These are soft and so fleshy that it is possible to nibble all the way round without biting into the itchy, hairy seeds. This makes the rose hips very easy to process. You can split them and scoop out the seeds rapidly in half the time of a dog rose. They are usually ready by the end of August/early September, though sometimes they can be quite plagued by worms, so you'll have to hunt for blemish-free fruit in a bad year.

Once you have deseeded the fruit you can either mash it with a blender, add the necessary sugar and process it into syrup or, to preserve all the good antioxidants and vitamin C, dry them in a dehydrator or somewhere warm and airy. Blend the dried fruit into a powder that can be sprinkled on top of breakfast muesli, on desserts or savoury foods or added to infusions for a winter hit of good stuff.

## How to grow

Dog rose, *R. canina*, is a rose of hedgerows and wild spaces that is native to the UK. It grows on scrubland, woodland edges and other sunny or dappled shaded spots in fertile ground. It's perhaps a little too wild and rambunctious for the garden. The Scottish or burnet rose, *R. pimpinellifolia*, is particularly pretty with ferny and delicate foliage and single flowers followed by currant-like black hips. The hips are a little hard to process and are best left whole, dried and then gently brought back to a slow simmer for tea, but it's a good rose for hedges, as it rarely grows taller than 1.5 m tall and can be persuaded to grow as ground cover. It has lovely pink flowers that in bud or open make for a wonderful tea and look very pretty dried. The sweet briar, *R. rubiginosa*, has wonderful apple-scented foliage and the young leaves when dried carefully impart this to other teas. The pink, highly scented flowers are equally good for teas. Both roses do well in poorer soils, but in general they favour fertility and dislike drying out. Once established roses are long-lived and very hard to kill. If you have an old bush that looks a little lacking, pour on well-rotted manure, shop-bought garden compost or anything from your own compost bin in autumn and prune hard, feeding again in spring.

As for rose pruning, this lot have evolved to be nibbled by hungry herbivores and rarely if ever are killed by a hard prune; however, flowering will be drastically reduced the following year if you hack everything back to ground level.

# How to use

Rose petals and rosebuds should be dried out of direct sunlight and turned regularly for even drying. Add these to any tea for a distinct floral note. I like them with black tea and a little lavender. This is quite delightful with honey on a hot afternoon or chilled and served with ice.

Rose hips can take up to a week to dry. This can be sped up in a dehydrator or on top of a radiator that is not too hot.

### For culinary use
For a particularly delicious rosehip syrup add ginger.

Rose water is made from distilling rose petals and you'll need a copper still for that. However, it's widely available from shops.

Rose petal vinegar needs to be made with very good-quality white wine vinegar. Fill a bottle with rose petals, then add the vinegar and store out of direct sunlight for 2 months, then strain and rebottle.

## Rose petal jam

Rose petal jam is a thing of beauty and works wonderfully with yoghurt. You'll need a bag of fresh small rose petals picked from plants free from pollution and pesticides.

250g small petals (*R. canina* is
   ideal)
450g granulated sugar

1.1 litres water
Juice 2 lemons

Place the petals in a bowl with half the sugar and leave overnight. This infuses the rose flavour into the sugar and darkens the petals.

In a heavy-based pan, add the water, lemon juice and remaining sugar, and then gently heat until all the sugar is dissolved. Stir in the rose petals and simmer for 20 minutes until the rose petals have softened. Turn the heat up and bring to a rapid boil for 5 minutes or until setting point is reached. Remove any scum that may have risen to the top and allow to cool slightly before stirring, so that the petals are evenly distributed. Cover and bottle. This jam should be fairly runny and not set hard, so that you can mix it like a compote into yoghurt.

# ROSEMARY

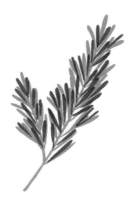

**Botanical Names** *Rosmarinus officinalis/Salvia rosamarinus.*

**Family** Lamiaceae (mint family).

**Parts Used** Flowers, twigs, leaves.

**Plant Properties** Carminative, antispasmodic, antidepressant, increases circulation, antimicrobial, increases menstrual flow.

**Uses** Sore throats, improves memory, calming effect on digestion, stimulates hair follicles and increases circulation to the scalp.

**Preparations** Culinary, infusions, teas.

**Considerations** Normal culinary amounts are fine, but large doses are not advised. Some people suffer from skin dermatitis when exposed to rosemary or its essential oil.

---

### The essential oil should be avoided in pregnancy and during breastfeeding.

---

R*os marinus* is Latin and means 'sea dew', for this is a plant that thrives on Mediterranean coasts where it can bake in the thin, well-drained, rocky soils and the gentle salt breeze concentrates its essential oils so that on a hot day you can smell the rosemary before you see it. Such a lovely romantic name then, until it was decided that rosemary doesn't sit in its own genus any more, but is actually a type of salvia and is much more closely linked to that other highly aromatic Mediterranean herb, sage. Still, I feel that this is one where we might just rebel against science and hold on to the more poetic Latin, for a while longer at least.

Rosemary is a powerful antimicrobial, particularly when used as an essential oil. It can be gargled or drunk as a calming, if rather powerful-tasting, tea to soothe sore throats. Rosemary is also very high in antioxidants and there are studies showing that it may prevent the formation of carcinogenic compounds in meat that is cooked on a high heat. Rosemary extract has also been shown to help treat UV damage to skin. The same antioxidants may also decrease oxidative stress (which is caused by an imbalance between the production of free radicals and the body's ability to counteract their effects) and inflammation, and therefore rosemary may have a role to play in reducing pain both as a topical and internal treatment. There have been some studies looking into rosemary's potential for arthritic pain.

In traditional folk medicine rosemary is the herb of remembrance and a sprig of the shrub is often used to symbolize a lost loved one at both weddings and funerals. It is also said that smelling rosemary will improve memory. Smelling a sprig of rosemary while studying and then again before an exam is said to improve your memory, and apparently this tradition goes as far back as ancient Greece. And the science suggests that there might be something in this. Smelling the essential oil of rosemary was said to reduce anxiety and significantly enhance memory. There's also some research into rosemary's effect on cognitive function in Alzheimer's patients.

Rosemary has a long history for digestive issues. Its anti-spasmodic and circulatory properties are said to gently stimulate the stomach and perhaps one reason it's been paired with fatty lamb and other meats is that it helps support the liver and digest fats.

Finally rosemary has a very long history for stimulating both hair follicles and the scalp, and may have some effect in treating premature baldness. It is said that rosemary essential oil is most beneficial for this process.

## How to grow

Rosemary loves to bask in the sun; it thrives in baked, free-draining soil. It will tolerate clay in the summer, but will hate the wet conditions that come in winter. If you want to grow rosemary in heavy soils, add plenty of grit to the plant hole and top-dress with grit too, so that it draws the water away from the crown. Rosemary can be grown in pots, but remember it wants to grow to a large shrub of 1 metre or more in height and cramming it into a 30cm pot is one way to make a miserable-looking bush. The prostrate form, *Salvia rosmarinus* 'Prostratus', lies flat to the ground and looks very handsome tumbling over a wall or down the sides of steps. Numerous other cultivars offer an array of sizes, flower colours and aromas. The standard upright types tend to be the best for culinary and medicinal purposes.

There is a fiendish beetle, known as the rosemary beetle, that wears a beautiful metallic green sheen on its wings. It's so good-looking you might think it a rather good addition to your rosemary plant, but it sucks the sap of the rosemary plant and can destroy it.

It will also destroy any neighbouring herbs, especially lavender, thyme and sage. The simplest way to get rid of the beetle is to pick it off.

# How to use

## Rosemary tea

Remove the twiggy stem and place 1 tablespoon of fresh rosemary leaves or 1 teaspoon of dried rosemary leaves in a cup. Bring 250ml of water to the boil and let it cool down; this is important as boiling water destroys some of the aromatic properties of rosemary. Pour over the leaves and cover for 5–10 minutes. I don't find it's necessary to strain as the rosemary tends to sink to the bottom of the cup. For sore throats and any other medicinal purposes, drink three times a day.

## Rosemary and sage hair wash

Regularly using rosemary on your hair will keep it shiny and your scalp conditioned. It will also darken your hair ever so gently. Sage will darken your hair even more quickly, and by combining the two and using every other day you'll see good results quite rapidly, even on grey hair. Once your hair has reached the desired colour use the wash once a week. If you have dark hair and want to see even better results, try adding 1 teaspoon of loose black tea to the mix.

I find it's easiest to make a tonic in a spray bottle and spray on to your hair after washing when still wet. You do not need to rinse it out.

4 cups water

8 tablespoons fresh chopped
   rosemary

8 tablespoons fresh chopped
   sage

Bring the water to a boil in a saucepan, then allow to cool to a simmer before adding the herbs. Simmer for 20 minutes, covered. Keep the lid on to allow the infused water to cool and then bottle. It's best if you can store this in the fridge as it eventually ferments. This will store for up to 2 months.

# RUE

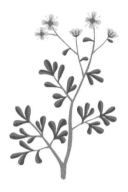

**Other Name**  Herb of grace.

**Botanical Name**  *Ruta graveolens.*

**Family**  Rutaceae (rue family).

**Parts Used**  Leaves.

**Plant Properties** Hepatotoxic, antispasmodic, antimicrobial, bitter, abortifacient, stimulates menstrual flow.

**Uses**  Medicinally used chiefly for its antispasmodic actions to relieve headache, relax griping and bowel tension, tension headaches and anxiety.

**Preparations**  Culinary.

**Considerations**  Large doses can cause gastric pain, vomiting, systemic complications and, in the worst-case scenario, death. Exposure to the sap or herbal preparations from it can cause phytophotodermatitis, including burn-like blisters on the skin. This happens when the sap is exposed to sun on the skin. When working in the garden around rue make sure to wear long sleeves and gloves, particularly if it is sunny. The essential oil is a very powerful abortifacient and therefore the plant should be avoided during pregnancy.

**Not to be used in pregnancy.**

Rue is a powerful herb with an ancient history as a medicine. The name 'Ruta' comes from the Greek word *reuo* and means to 'set free', referring to its reputation for freeing people from disease. It's far too strong a herb for the amateur to attempt to use, but one for the wise, qualified practitioner. However, if you have got this far in my alphabet, you will have found all sorts of idiosyncrasies, oddities and whims, and although rue is potentially dangerous it is also delicious and deserves exploring.

The plant is often associated with the verb 'rue', meaning to regret or be sorrowful. It's from this that it gets its name as the herb of grace, giving a symbolic meaning to regret. Ophelia in *Hamlet* (Act IV, Scene 5) strews flowers in grief-stricken madness, '. . . there's rue for you, and here's some for me; we may call it herb of grace o' Sundays; O, you must wear your rue with a difference', suggesting both regret, but also that the herb was used to treat pain and maybe even something to do with the herb's abortive qualities.

Rue is native to the Balkan peninsula, but is now grown worldwide perhaps in recognition of its medicinal importance in years gone by. It's a strange-looking plant with bluish leaves and bright yellow flowers. It is deeply tolerant of hot and dry soil conditions and loves a long, baking summer and hugely hates our damp winters.

Although no one could claim rue is widely used in culinary terms, those regions that use it do so passionately. It was frequently used in Roman cuisine and it is said that chewing on a few of the fresh leaves will relieve tension headaches, ease palpitations and alleviate many other anxiety problems.

In northern Italy and Istria, in Croatia, it is used to flavour grappa or raki. The seed can be used in porridge. In Friuli-Venezia Guilia in Italy whole young branches are dipped in batter, deep-fried and then consumed with sugar and salt. They are also used to make a type of omelette.

It's hard to pinpoint the exact flavour of rue, but if you were to think of it as the Mediterranean version of lemongrass and use it as such, you'd have a starting point. It is a sour, bitter herb and needs to be used sparingly for best effect.

# How to grow

*Ruta graveolens* is a small, semi-woody shrub growing up to 60cm tall and 75cm wide. In a sheltered position it is often evergreen, but when exposed to frosts or cold winds it will drop all its leaves. The much-loved cultivar 'Jackman's Blue' has dainty foliage, almost like that of a maidenhair fern, with a metallic blue-green bloom to the leaves that is most obvious in full sun.

Seeds should be sown from March to May in a propagator very shallowly. Do not cover them with compost as they need light to germinate. Make sure the compost is damp but not wet. The best results come if the seed tray is covered with a propagator lid or sealed in a polythene bag until germination. This can take up to twenty-one days at 20°C/68°F. Plant them out into their permanent position after the last frost. Once your plant is established you may find it self-seeds, so deadhead if this is a bother.

# How to use

## For culinary use

Use the leaves sparingly with eggs, cheese or meats. Start with an omelette and experiment from there. A traditional recipe of damson plums in red wine is flavoured with rue to add to meat. Rue can also be added to spicy Italian tomato sauces just towards the end of cooking, but should be removed before serving. It can be added to pickled vegetables, herbal vinegar and salads.

# SAGE

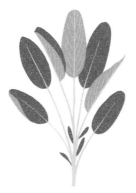

**Botanical Name** *Salvia officinalis.*
**Family** Lamiaceae (mint family).
**Parts Used** Leaves, flowers.
**Plant Properties** Antiviral, antibacterial, antimicrobial, antifungal, astringent, anti-inflammatory.
**Uses** For sore throats, for mouthwash and gum health, scalp tonic.
**Preparations** Hair/scalp tonics, infusions, teas, toothpaste.

**Considerations** Sage contains a chemical compound known as thujone and doses of 15g or more can cause tachycardia (an elevated heart rate at rest), hot flushes, convulsions and dizziness. It is very important not to use any leaves that are mildewed for cooking or medicinal consumption.

**Should be avoided in pregnancy, except as a culinary spice.**

Everyone ends up with too much sage, for once you've browned some butter with sage for gnocchi or stuffed some pork belly with the stuff, what are you supposed to do with so many leaves? Make *uccelli scappati* for one thing. *Uccelli scappati* translates as 'the runaway birds' or 'the birds that have flown'. Take two of the largest sage leaves you can find, place between them a little bit of anchovy or anchovy paste, dip in batter and fry in very hot oil. Allow briefly to cool before eating with either a very cold glass of wine or a good beer. You can substitute the anchovy for a little sliver of hard cheese for a vegetarian version. Quite delicious.

Still, even *uccelli scappati* might not use up all your sage leaves. Garden sage, *Salvia officinalis*, has powerful antibacterial properties and has long been used to fight infections. It was an early kind of toothpaste and is known to promote good gum health. It has been used to treat gingivitis and mouth ulcers. Taken internally, sage is said to be a good carminative, relieving flatulence, and is said to decrease sweating and dry up breast milk production during weaning.

# How to grow

Sage loves hot, dry conditions and does best in full sun. In shade it can get mildew, particularly if there is poor air circulation. Sage is known to get woody and have rather unsightly bare legs. To prevent this cut back the plant hard after flowering to new growth, but never into the woody stems without sign of life, as it rarely responds well to that.

It's very easy to take cuttings of sage. Take semi-ripe cuttings that are 10–15 cm long between August and September. The stem should be firm at the base and soft at the tip. Discard both the tip and the firm base so that you are left with the middle section. Cut just below the leaf node and pinch out the bottom two sets of leaves. You should have two sets of leaves left; insert these into seed compost round the edge of the pot and cover with a clear plastic bag. Make sure the cuttings are left somewhere warm but out of direct sunlight; a windowsill is usually perfect. They will root quickly. You can also root sage directly in water the same way.

There are numerous cultivars of sage, including 'Purpurascens', a purple-leafed form; 'Tricolor' a pink, white and green form; 'Elephant Ear', an elongated large-leafed form; and 'Common Broad Leaf' form, which has wider leaves.

## Sage tea/infusion

Put 1–2 teaspoons of fresh leaves in 1 cup (250ml) of boiling water, cover and leave to stand for 10 minutes. This can be drunk up to three times a day.

You can make a mouthwash using the same method, but use 2 teaspoons of fresh leaves in 500ml of water and gargle warm or cold as you prefer.

## Sage flower pesto

If your sage flowers well, collect the sticky flowers just after opening and make a pesto with them. The flowers are sweeter than the leaves, but still have a pronounced sage flavour. You'll need to pick 30 or more flowers for a pesto with a little garlic, pine or walnuts, olive oil and parmesan. This works particularly well on pasta or gnocchi.

## Sage toothpaste

I first read about this method from the wonderful Juliette de Baïracli Levy, aka *Juliette of the Herbs*, and made some out of curiosity in the hope that it would use up the mountains of sage I grow. Now I have to admit that I love the flavour so much that I am as likely to sprinkle it on my food (it's wonderful over roasting potatoes) as I am my teeth.

Take fresh sage leaves and place them on a baking tray at 180°C/350°F. Bake for a few minutes until crisp. Keep an eye on them as they turn quickly, and you don't want a single burnt edge.

In a clean coffee grinder or pestle and mortar grind the sage to a fine powder with sea salt to taste. There's no prescribed amount of sea salt here, but you want a scant handful of coarse sea salt to a tray of baked leaves. The desired effect is that the paste is salty, but not too much so.

Use this once a week as a toothpaste. The mixture is quite abrasive and, unless your coffee grinder is particularly good, you'll want to use the sage salt rub first, rinse and then use your regular toothpaste or else you'll find little bits of sage stuck between your teeth.

Salt rinses are known to help with bad breath, to fight gingivitis and reduce inflammation. The astringent effects of sage help to tighten gums and prevent the bacteria commonly found in plaque, *Streptococcus mutans*, which is a significant contributor to tooth decay.

Store the sage/salt rub in an airtight container and keep somewhere cool. It will store for many months this way.

# SAVORY

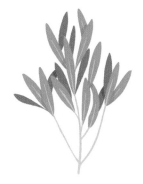

**Botanical Names** *Satureja hortensis* (summer savory), *Satureja montana* (winter savory).

**Family** Lamiaceae (mint family).

**Parts Used** Fresh or dried leaves and stems.

**Plant Properties** Astringent, aromatic, expectorant, stomach-soothing, improves digestion, carminative, antiseptic, antioxidant.

**Uses** For colds, for insect stings, increases circulation, to relieve flatulence and bloating.

**Preparations** Culinary spice; poultices for insect stings; salves; teas.

**Considerations** None known.

The peppery tang of summer savory ensures there's no doubt about where it gets its name from; it truly is the most savoury herb of the culinary spices. It is widely used in Romanian and Bulgarian dishes and is one of the characteristic ingredients of *herbes de Provence* and is known for its natural affinity with beans; this is in part because it is a very good carminative, stimulating the digestion and eliminating gas. It has a cousin, winter savory, but with its hardiness comes a bitter note, which means that for culinary purposes summer savory is always favoured.

It is often dried for winter use and its peppery notes are even more pronounced this way. Recipes vary but in cuisines and households where it is loved it is often used by the generous spoonful and it's well worth experimenting with it in sauces, stews, meat marinades and rubs. Think of it as a spicier sage with a hint of thyme and mint.

# How to grow

Summer savory is an annual and is not frost-hardy. I find the seeds can be very slow to germinate and nearly always start the plant off indoors on a heated propagator mat, pricking out the seedlings when they are large enough to handle into individual modules. When the plant is 10cm high or so I pinch out the tops to encourage branching. Only the tender young stems and leaves should be used in cooking because they impart the most flavour and are least likely to have soil splash-back, where the rain hits the soil and splashes it on to the leaves, giving them a gritty taste if not washed thoroughly. I find that they do best either in pots in good peat-free compost or in a very sunny position in well-drained soil in the garden. Savory plants will sulk if grown in the shade. Traditionally when the plant starts to flower in August the whole thing is pulled up to dry.

Winter savory is a perennial herb of much hardier conditions. It is evergreen and available all year round, has considerably fewer essential oils and is far coarser, but in winter it makes a decent substitute if the dried summer savory has run out. Again, it prefers free-draining conditions in a sunny position where it will grow into a low, slow-spreading mound.

# How to use

## Savory tea
Tea of fresh or dried leaves can be drunk freely, makes a good after-dinner tisane, can be used to treat sore throats and may be gargled with. Use 1 tablespoon of the fresh herb, or 1 teaspoon of dried herb, with 250ml of boiling water, and steep for 10 minutes, covered.

## For medicinal use
Medicinally savory is used in several ways. The most common is to aid digestion as a tea. It can be combined with other herbs, such as caraway or fennel, where it will add a peppery note to an after-dinner tisane.

It can also be used as a poultice for stings and bites. The easiest way to do this is to mash the fresh herb, in your mouth if necessary, and place over the sting, where it will immediately help to relieve pain and reduce swelling, or it can be made into a salve or oil for massaging into the skin, where it has a warming effect and is said to stimulate the circulation.

## Savory salve
A herbal oil of summer savory is easy to make by infusing the dried or fresh herb in oil, leaving somewhere warm in a sunny position, then straining and rebottling. The oil can be used for massages and for this reason it's best to either use olive, jojoba or almond oil. For fresh herbs you need a ratio of one to three; for dried herbs you need a ratio of one to five, so 100g of dried herb to 500ml of olive, jojoba or almond oil.

100g summer savory leaves        300ml olive, jojoba or
                                    almond oil

Finely mince the leaves, place in a clean jar and cover with oil. Stir thoroughly to remove any air bubbles. When the time comes to remove the herbs, pour through several layers of muslin and squeeze the herbs to further express the oil.

As fresh herbs still contain a lot of water this will end up being extracted into the oil as sludge. It is necessary to drain this off otherwise the oil may spoil. Leave the mixture overnight and the sludgy particulate matter and water will settle to the bottom of the jar. Carefully pour off the clear oil from the top into a new bottle and discard the sludge. Store the finished herbal oil in a clean, tightly stoppered bottle or jar.

It is very important that the plant material is completely covered by the oil or it will be exposed to microbes in the air, turning it mouldy. Air bubbles should be removed for the same reason. Seal the jar and leave somewhere warm in the sun. Turn the jar daily to ensure even sun distribution. After 2 weeks the oil should have extracted the plant's essence.

This process can be sped up by putting the oil in a bain-marie or slow cooker. You will need to simmer the oil for 2–3 hours.

Once the oil is infused strain out the plant material. You can make a stronger solution at this point by adding new fresh herbs and repeating the process.

If stored in a cool dry place, the oil will keep for up to a year.

# SELFHEAL

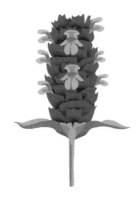

**Other Names** Heal-all, common selfheal, woundwort, heart-of-the-earth, carpenter's herb, brownwort.
**Botanical Name** *Prunella vulgaris*.
**Family** Lamiaceae (mint family).
**Parts Used** Leaves, flowers, young stems.

**Plant Properties** Astringent, styptic, antimicrobial, bitter, diuretic.
**Uses** Cuts and wounds, boils and bruises, mouth ulcers, sore throats.
**Preparations** Poultices, teas.
**Considerations** None known.

Selfheal, as the name suggests, is a powerful herb traditionally used for stemming bleeding and promoting the healing of cuts, wounds and mouth ulcers. It can help with heavy periods and as a cream for haemorrhoids. You are most likely to find this herb growing in your lawn for it's a low-growing wildflower of grassland and fields, happy to creep just below the mower blades and take a risk at flowering every once in a while. All my life I have known that if you mash the leaves up in your mouth and apply them under a plaster to nasty grazes or stubborn wounds on knuckles and joints they will start to heal overnight and begin to knit together. Its other name is carpenter's herb, but I think it's just as apt for gardeners who suffer too many pruning saw scrapes and thorn-punctured cuts.

# How to grow

This is a common wildflower; any park or wildish lawn will have some poking about. The plant grows to no more than 10cm high and has distinct square stems characteristic of its family, with small opposite lanceolate leaves. The flower spike is borne just above the top two leaves, so that they appear to wrap round it like a collar; the flower spike has typical Lamiaceae hooded flowers in blue-purple whorls. It prefers sunny to part-shade conditions and likes to be fairly damp.

# How to use

## For medicinal use

An infusion of the leaves and flowers can be used to gargle with for mouth ulcers or sore throats. Use 2 tablespoons of leaves and flowers in 250ml of boiling water, covered for 10 minutes to steep and then allowed to cool so you can gargle with it. For sore throats it's possible to combine honey with cold tea – one part tea to two parts honey – to make a syrup to soothe the throat.

## Selfheal poultice

Macerate the leaves, young stems and flowers until they release their juices. Pack this mixture on to a cleaned wound and cover with gauze or a plaster and leave overnight. In the morning replace with a new poultice. The juice of the macerated material can also be used to stem bleeding as a styptic. Clearly this is only suitable for minor wounds.

# SORREL

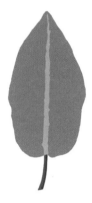

**Other Names** Garden sorrel, common sorrel.

**Botanical Name** *Rumex acetosa.*

**Family** Polygonaceae (knotweed family).

**Parts Used** Leaves, stems, seeds.

**Plant Properties** Nutritive, appetite-stimulant, antimicrobial, anti-inflammatory, astringent, antioxidant.

**Uses** To help reduce fever and infections; a vitamin and mineral boost.

**Preparations** Culinary.

**Considerations** Sorrel contains oxalic acid and eating too much can prevent the uptake of minerals like calcium and magnesium; it is also a no-go for anyone with kidney stones. When cooking sorrel add sour cream or milk to chelate the oxalic acid; this binds the oxalic acid with calcium, making it insoluble, so it passes harmlessly through the digestive system. Drinking plenty of water will also help.

The lemon zest of a sorrel leaf, reminiscent of the sour tang of unripe wild strawberries or hard kiwi fruit, tells you that this plant is packed with vitamin C. On top of that sorrel has a great whack of vitamin A, as well as good amounts of many B-complex vitamins and minerals, such as manganese, zinc, copper and potassium. It was once widely used against scurvy and has a folk history for its use against stomach ulcers due to its anti-inflammatory and antioxidant (that's the copper and manganese, which acts as a cofactor for the antioxidant enzyme superoxide dismutase) properties. There have been limited scientific studies on this, but there is some evidence that it has a positive role to play in anti-ulcer activity in mice, particularly if it is extracted in alcohol.

Sorrel is often left off or barely mentioned in herbals, but it seems a shame when it's such a delicious and easy herb to grow. I'm not suggesting if you have an ulcer that you should suddenly eat lots of the stuff, but I do think everyone should be adding this one to their salads. It's a daily vitamin dose that is very palatable, and sorrel is often up and green when there are few other salads to be picking in early spring. Plus, the slugs don't touch it and it's perennial, so there's very little work in growing it. You find its happy place in your garden and then you eat it, that's it.

## How to grow

Sheep's sorrel, *Rumex acetosella*, grows wild in damp, marshy places and tends to have small (up to 3cm long) leaves. Then there's garden sorrel, *R. acetosa*, which has long, leathery leaves. French sorrel or buckler-leaved sorrel, *R. scutatus*, has shield-shaped leaves up to 10cm long, is pale green in colour, and is slightly less sour than garden sorrel.

All sorrels like to grow in well-drained but rich soils in sun or lightly shaded spots. They hate to dry out in summer, but have long, deep taproots, so once they become established they tend to seek out their own water. Young plants will need to be watered regularly in dry periods and they need a large pot so that the roots can roam to be happy. Often they try to flower regularly through the summer. The flower spike can grow to over 1 metre tall and is covered in tiny pink flowers and eventually thousands of seeds. To prevent it diverting all its energy to seeds rather than leaves, nip out the spike before it starts to flower. However, if you've found the plant has already bolted to flowering, don't waste the blooms, which hold a sweeter version of the lemony tang of the leaves and can be sprinkled over salads or added to dressings. 'Profusion' is a non-flowering form that shoots many more leaves and is well worth looking out for.

After several years you may find that your sorrel has become quite woody in the middle and endlessly flowers. When this happens divide the plant in spring or autumn and replant with some well-rotted garden compost. You can sow from February to July, but you will have to sow indoors to get good germination if planting earlier in the year. From May onwards you can sow direct, thinning seedlings so that plants are around 20cm apart. Three plants are plenty for most.

# How to use

## For culinary use

The leaf and stem can be eaten raw in salads or briefly cooked. Sorrel sauce is lovely on fish. Reduce some stock by half – you can add a minced shallot in, if you like, or a little vermouth, then add cream, salt and pepper, and when ready to serve add a handful of finely chopped sorrel and stir in.

Sorrel also works well when combined with sour cream for a dip. There are many versions of sorrel soup, with vegetables, herbs, meat or eggs. It is also often mixed in with spinach, used in curries and as a filling for pies. The high oxalic acid content means that you shouldn't eat too much of this herb, but its incredibly sour flavour will naturally limit how much you consume.

# ST JOHN'S WORT

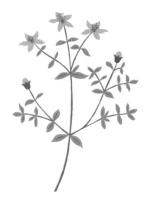

**Other Names** Common St John's wort, perforate St John's wort.

**Botanical Name** *Hypericum perforatum.*

**Family** Hypericaceae (St John's wort family).

**Parts Used** Flowering and budding tops, roughly the top 10cm of the plant.

**Plant Properties** Anti-inflammatory, astringent, nervine, antimicrobial, wound-healing.

**Uses** Salve for sprains, swelling, old burns, minor wounds.

**Preparations** Infusions, oils, teas.

**Considerations** Not to be taken alongside pharmaceutical drugs. May cause photosensitivity particularly if taken in large doses. In large quantities St John's wort is poisonous to grazing livestock.

**Not to be used while pregnant or breastfeeding, or for small children.**

St John's wort's antidepressant properties are well known; it has been used for centuries to treat mental health problems and sleep disorders and today has been proven by some studies to help mild to moderate depression. Research suggests that it increases the activity of brain chemicals such as serotonin and noradrenaline. Its chief components are hypericin and hyperforin, but the plant contains many other substances that are thought to act as antidepressants which are not currently fully understood. However, it is always important to point out that St John's wort is not to be taken concurrently with pharmaceutical drugs, such as oral contraceptives, antihistamines, certain antibiotics and antifungals among others. Nor should it replace antidepressants without first seeking help from your doctor.

Perhaps less well known are St John's wort's incredible anti-inflammatory and wound-healing properties. The use of red oil made from its flowers and unopened buds for healing bruises, sprains and mild burns can be traced back to the Crusades, which is where it is thought to have got its name from, as it was used by the Knights Hospitaller, the order of St John. It is also supposed to be incredibly effective for healing sunburn and is a great pain reliever for shingles.

St John's Day is on 24 June and celebrates the feast of St John the Baptist; it's also when you traditionally harvest St John's wort.

## How to grow

*Hypericum perforatum* is a wild flower of Europe and Asia, but is now grown worldwide. It is often found growing in scrubby wasteland in full sun. It is considered a noxious weed in many parts of the world. Once you have an eye for it, particularly its yolk-yellow flowers in midsummer, you'll start spotting it everywhere. This is a plant I would forage for rather than introduce into my garden. It grows up to 1 metre tall and has opposite stalkless, narrow oblong leaves at 1–2cm long, which are scattered with translucent glandular dots. If held to the light the leaf looks perforated, hence its specific epithet, *perforatum*. The flowers are bright yellow with conspicuous black dots; there are many stamens that are united at the base into three bundles. The flowers appear at the end of the upper branches from late spring to midsummer. The flower bud when bruised, or the seeds when crushed, give a reddish/purple dye, hence the colour of red oil.

# How to use

When picking flowers and flower buds to dry or use fresh it is important that you pick the top 10cm of the plant and include some of the leaves. The leaves contain active flavonoids, plant pigments that are said to enhance the activity of the hypericin found in the flowers and buds. The flowers are best picked in midsummer. The hypericin is readily absorbed when picking the flowers, so when processing large batches wear gloves and long sleeves and wash any exposed parts with soap and water to prevent photosensitivity. Do not rub your eyes.

### St John's wort tea

The flowers and buds can be used fresh or dried for tea. Use 1 teaspoon of dried herb per 250ml of water, or 1 tablespoon of fresh flowers/buds, and drink up to three times a day. Please remember to talk to a medical healthcare professional before taking St John's wort internally as it interacts with many prescription medicines.

## Red oil

Only fresh flowers and buds can be used to make red oil. Use 1 part herb by volume to 3 parts of olive oil. Allow the flowers and buds to wilt slightly and then mash or bruise them thoroughly before placing them in a rubber-sealed preservation jar and topping up with olive oil. Don't strip the flowers from the stem, because this helps to stop the mash becoming too clumped together. Leave the jar in the sun for 2 weeks to macerate. Then strain and rebottle, keeping the oil out of direct sunlight. It should keep for a year.

Use the oil externally as needed for inflammation, nerve pain, bruises and minor cuts and burns.

# SWEET VIOLET

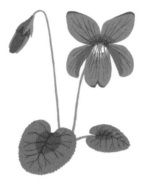

**Other Names** Violet, heartsease.

**Botanical Names** *Viola odorata* (sweet violet), *Viola tricolor* (heartsease).

**Family** Violaceae (violet family).

**Parts Used** Fresh or dried aerial portions of the plant picked in early-flowering stages, including the stems, leaves and flowers.

**Plant Properties** Anti-inflammatory, emollient, expectorant.

**Uses** Skin disorders, coughs and upper respiratory infections, bruises.

**Preparations** Poultices, salves, teas, washes.

**Considerations** Should be avoided by those with an allergy to salicylic acid.

I f you find a patch big enough, the heavenly Parma violet smell will give it away in spring. For such a tiny plant sweet violet, *Viola odorata*, packs a punch with its perfume. It loves dappled shade, such as a spot under a deciduous tree or on a damp bank, and if left undisturbed will produce a great bank of delightful purple flowers. It is the first of the violets to flower in spring, followed by the scentless dog violet, *V. riviniana* and then by heartsease, *V. tricolor*. *V. odorata* is considered a stronger medicine in herbalism than heartsease or the common dog violet. Other than its unmistakable scent, the sweet violet is recognizable by its sprays of violet or white flowers, blunt sepals and creeping stolons. The flowers appear from February to May. When the seed is set in June it is often spread by ants, who are fond of the sticky, fleshy structure on the seed, known as an elaiosome, and will carry them for some distance. The seed can remain dormant in the soil for some years waiting for the right conditions, which is why they seemingly spring up out of nowhere in slightly neglected, mossy lawns.

## How to grow

*V. odorata* grows in moist soil in partial shade and will work well in a pot too. If its soil is damp enough, it will tolerate full sun. If growing in a pot, try getting hold of an alpine pan, a wide, shallow pot for alpine flowers, which will give it space to spread. The seed should be sown in autumn as it seems to do best with a long cold period to break dormancy; a second sowing can be made in early spring. You can sow direct or in modules to plant out in mid- to late spring. Each plant will eventually spread to 30cm, but they don't mind mingling together and working it out, so plant 15cm apart. They work well under shrubs and deciduous trees, but also make an excellent ground cover under roses and are good for north-facing aspects.

# How to use

Pick the aerial portions of the plant, including stems and leaves, in the early-flowering stage.

## Sweet violet tea

Use 1 teaspoon of dried or 1 tablespoon of fresh herb and infuse for 10 minutes, covered. This tea can be drunk up to three times a day for coughs and other minor upper respiratory conditions.

## For medicinal use

You can make a poultice of freshly mashed or bruised leaves, flowers and stems, which is said to be very good for healing and drawing out infections.

The herb has a long-standing use as a cough remedy and makes a gentle floral tea that is safe enough for children (if you can get them to drink such a thing). It can also be used for skin conditions and is reputedly good for eczema. The tea is often prescribed for urinary tract infections. You can make a herbal oil using the same method as for calendula (see page 175) and this is good for moisturizing and toning the skin.

# Other species

Heartsease, *Viola tricolor*, has an equally long history for coughs, bronchitis and other upper respiratory conditions. Much like sweet violet, it has been used for skin conditions, including eczema and cradle cap in babies. The herb is often cited for cystitis; this is because it contains both salicylates and rutin, which are anti-inflammatory. Heartsease is mildly laxative and some herbalists believe it to be gentler than *Viola odorata*. As *Viola tricolor* has little scent, the tea is a little duller, but can be drunk in the same quantities and it's certainly a good addition to any tea to keep coughs at bay.

# TARRAGON

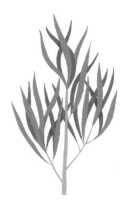

**Other Name** Estragon.

**Botanical Name** *Artemisia dracunculus.*

**Family** Asteraceae (sunflower or daisy family).

**Parts Used** Leaves, soft stems.

**Plant Properties** Aromatic, warming, improves digestion, diuretic, appetite-stimulant, reduces fever, mildly sedative.

**Uses** Reduces pain of toothache, aids digestion, relieves bloating and flatulence, lowers fever, aids sleep.

**Preparations** Culinary.

**Considerations** None known.

---

**Not to be used by pregnant women.**

---

Never fall for Russian tarragon; its looks are deceptively similar, but it all ends there. Russian tarragon, *Artemisia dracunculoides*, is coarse and frankly flavourless compared to French tarragon, which is grassy, herbal and with a distinct note of anise and vanilla to its fine soft leaves. Russian tarragon is very hardy and vigorous and people tend to be swayed by that.

Tarragon is most associated with French cuisine, which holds it so dear to its heart and its Béarnaise sauce. Tarragon vinegar, a chief component of said sauce, is also a very good way to store leaves over winter when the plant dies back. Tarragon is often paired with mushrooms, fish, egg and chicken. It also makes a great addition to fermented pickles and is often used in Persian-style pickles, particularly cucumber ones. It is a popular component of a sugary fizzy drink in Armenia, Azerbaijan, Georgia, Russia, the Ukraine and Kazakhstan. The drink, in my experience, is incredibly sweet and a violent neon green.

Tarragon has a medicinal folk history; though, like savory, you don't see it mentioned much these days. It makes a very good digestive tea, helping to relieve bloating, flatulence, hiccups and nausea, and is mildly sedative, so perfect for after dinner when it works nicely combined with Korean mint. Traditionally a poultice was made from its fresh leaves and used to help with toothache. It is also said to reduce both the pain and length of a fever.

## How to grow

Tarragon loves free-draining conditions and dislikes a cold, wet winter. It seems to be most long-lived in poorer soils and dislikes clay. It also dislikes being crowded out and needs full sun. I've had the best success growing it in a pot with lots of grit added to the potting compost (up to half in volume) and top-dressed with more grit. Once established it is very drought-tolerant and can cope with intermittent watering. French tarragon does not set viable seed and so you will have to buy a young plant. In a pot the plant will last for around three years, by which time it will start to get tired and unproductive. Taking cuttings is quite hard and it's usually easiest to either use the underground runners to take root cuttings or divide the plant every two years or so to keep it productive; this should be done in spring.

# How to use

## For culinary use

Nothing beats fresh tarragon. You won't need much – a sprig or two straight from your garden will provide plenty of flavour. Towards the end of summer I tend to cut the whole plant back and add to good-quality white wine vinegar to flavour. This takes 2 weeks, but I generally just leave the herb in place in the vinegar rather than straining.

## For medicinal use

A tea can be made of the fresh or dried herb to relieve bloating, nausea, hiccups and flatulence. Use 1 teaspoon of dried herb or 1 tablespoon of fresh herb to 250ml of boiling water, then cover and allow to steep for 10 minutes before serving with honey, if preferred.

It works well mixed with either liquorice mint, garden mint, dried apple, lemon peel and green tea or a combination of these.

# THISTLES

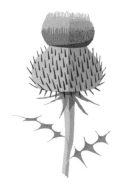

**Botanical Names** *Sonchus* species, *Lactua muralis, Silybum marianum.*
**Family** Asteraceae (sunflower or daisy family).
**Parts Used** Seeds, leaves.
**Plant Properties** Anti-inflammatory, antioxidant, antiviral, nutritive.
**Uses** Protects liver (milk thistle), nutritive (sow thistle, wall lettuce).
**Preparations** Culinary.
**Considerations** None known.

Apale apple-green with a bluish sheen to the leaves, the stem as thick as my thumb, perhaps the first hint of flower: that is a perfect sow thistle to eat. It's a tricky business, though. Not only for the spines, spikes and prickles – those are obvious hurdles to be removed – but the peeling of the stem. For the outer stem of thistle is tough and so bitter as to leave your mouth puckered, but the inside, if caught at the right moment, is so delicious. A hint of nuttiness, a tempered bitter, a good crunch, like a celery, but with clout. When I see a perfect sow thistle I can think only of peeling the stem to get to all that goodness. And it was the sow thistle more than any other plant that taught me the pleasure of truly listening and responding to my body. That grazing like a herbivore through the garden, eating what my body craved rather than a recipe suggests, is a very good way to take your medicine.

Sow thistles are two a dozen and available nearly all year round; you can spot them in the depths of winter or the height of summer growing where they find the best position – in shade in summer, in full sun in winter, as is the wont and speed of a weed. And I do not always look at them and want to instantly eat them, but when I do get that craving I know my body is in need of their specific nutritive tonic.

Many of the herbs in this book fall into the browsing category. If you have a sudden desire to eat sorrel in spring or crave the heat of rocket in autumn, if you can't get enough of the first blackberries and find yourself on a detour to take more in, if the dandelions you are weeding out look suddenly very appealing in all their lush growth, don't compost them; instead, nibble on them.

There are three groups of thistles that I either grow or welcome as weeds. The first is the wall lettuce, *Lactua muralis*, which is a weed of roadsides, walls, gardens, field margins, rocky areas and woodland edges, usually on chalk or limestone soil. It's the one you might find out on a weekend walk in the countryside or city limits. Wall lettuce is found all over the UK and is similar-looking to the sow thistle, but has distinct purple-tinged basal leaves. The stem leaves have deep, large-toothed, squarish lobes with red-tinged ribs and small yellow flowers – not a million miles away from a dandelion, except the whole plant is blueish green. The leaves are used in salads and have a more delicate, less bitter taste than the sow thistle.

## The sow thistles

There are three in this gang: the perennial sow thistle, *Sonchus arvensis*, the prickly sow thistle, *S. asper*, and the smooth sow thistle, *S. oleraceus*. All three are edible, though without doubt the smooth sow-thistle is the best-tasting and the one you find most commonly as an opportunistic invader of open soil in gardens, fields, cliff edges, pavements and roadsides. It has hollow stems and a long history of being used as a leafy green vegetable.

All three look to some extent like dandelions and also bear a superficial resemblance to true thistles, though they lack sharp thistles. They have dandelion-like flower heads, but these grow in clusters from the main leafy stem, unlike the dandelion, which has a single flower stem. *S. oleraceus* is an annual herb with a hollow upright stem up to 100cm high, but normally 30cm or so. The leaves are dullish grey-green and lobed without prickles. Its flowers are pale yellow and small, up to 20mm wide. The seeds tend to germinate in autumn to spring and produce a rosette of leaves. Later the plant produces a milky stem with close-growing larger, glossier leaves.

*S. oleraceus* is the one to go on the hunt for. It has such a long history as a wild edible that there's considerable research on its nutritive qualities. It is rich in vitamin C, beta-carotene and protein. It also has appreciable amounts of vitamin A and calcium. It has a long history of use among Maoris, who said it would make a person grow strong. In herbalism it is considered to have similar properties to dandelion and chicory, and makes an excellent spring tonic. It is a folkloric solution to warts. It certainly makes for a delicious wild green that can be used like you might spinach or chard if cooked, or raw like an endive or bitter green, with far more vitamins and minerals than any of its cultivated counterparts can offer. It is sometimes called a milk thistle due to its white sap, but if you are looking for the best liver tonic, then you need the true milk thistle, *Silybum marianum*.

## Milk thistle

The milk thistle is the true herb of hangovers. It has a long, well-reputed history as a liver tonic and this characteristic is increasingly being recognized in the latest research, which shows that the constituents of milk thistle protect liver cells from chemical damage. Milk thistle seeds contain silymarin, which is a group of flavonoids (including silibinin, silidianin and silicristin) that are known to help repair cells when they've been damaged by toxins. These flavonoids can also help protect new liver cells. While all parts of the plants are edible, only the seeds contain appreciable amounts of silymarin.

# How to grow

Milk thistle is a stout biennial that grows up to 1 metre tall with branched stems crowned in several light purple flowers. They tend to flower from June to August. The leaves are oblong to lanceolate in shape, either lobed or pinnate with incredibly spiny edges. The leaves have very distinct milky-white veins and the upper leaves clasp the stem. It's distinctly thistle-looking and the milky-white venation makes it instantly recognizable. It grows wild all over the UK, but I think it plenty handsome enough for the garden and the bees love it. In its first year of flowering I suggest only harvesting half the seeds and letting the rest scatter about. If it likes you, it may quickly colonize the space. It prefers dry, well-drained soils and, surprisingly for all those lethal spines, can get munched by slugs if not protected. It is possible to grow in a pot and makes quite a striking specimen if grown in clumps in large pots (30cm diameter plus). It is often found growing in waste ground and is found worldwide as a weed. If you are going to harvest on a large scale, you'll need plenty of space. The seed heads are very attractive over winter, but to harvest the seed efficiently you'll need to chop them off to process, so bear that in mind when you place them in your midsummer garden, because you'll have a bit of a bare hole later in the year.

## How to use

Milk thistle is harvested mostly for its seeds, which are collected when mature and dry. The thistles on this plant are brutal; you must wear gloves to do this. Seeds appear quickly after the flower has finished blooming and the easiest way to process them is to cut off the flower head. A good healthy flower head produces numerous seeds that taste bitter but not unpleasant.

Perhaps the easiest way to take milk thistle seed is to grind it up and consume it directly. It can be sprinkled on cereal or added to yoghurt. The milled seed will go rancid quickly, though it can be stored in a fridge for a couple of days. Therefore it's best to grind the seed as needed. It is recommended to take 12–15g of seeds a day, which is roughly 2 tablespoons. It is said that this is especially beneficial for anyone living or working around polluted environments. If you are going out drinking, try taking milk thistle seed beforehand and again the morning after. You can chew the seeds if you prefer.

# THYME

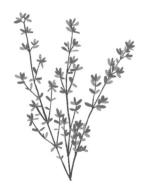

**Other Name** Common thyme.

**Botanical Name** *Thymus vulgaris*.

**Family** Lamiaceae (mint family).

**Parts Used** Dried or fresh leaves and soft young stems.

**Plant Properties** Astringent, antiseptic, aromatic, carminative, deodorant, expectorant, sedative, tonic, antimicrobial, antifungal.

**Uses** Coughs, indigestion, fungal infections, sore throats and respiratory conditions.

**Preparations** Culinary, moth repellent, teas.

**Considerations** Medicinal amounts of thyme and thyme essential oil should not be used by pregnant women; large amounts of thyme are not recommended when breastfeeding either.

If you have ever been in the Mediterranean on an afternoon so warm that you smell the thyme before you even brush up against it, then you know that it thrives in rocky outcroppings in earth so thin that it is hard to call it soil. If you've grown thyme in the UK, though, you'll know that it can grow in damp, rich soil too; though you

274

shouldn't expect to have a long relationship with your thyme plant. It will be with you and then it won't . . . Just like that.

Thyme is best suited to a garden path's edge. Shingle, brick or similar will allow it to drain freely and creep around as it wishes. If your soil is in the least bit heavy, add plenty of grit. The thyme wants to sit in a pocket of the stuff and don't ever imagine that it wants even a hint of shade.

Thyme is legendary in the kitchen and forms the basis of so many dishes. Its fragrant, sweet, strong herbaceous notes with a hint of mint, lemon and pepper are robust enough to withstand long, slow cooking. It is the perfect match for slow-stewed tomatoes; it cuts through the fat of lamb to bring the pasture notes of dairy alive; it sits well with pork; and is delicious just soaked in olive oil.

As a herbal medicine thyme is prized for its antimicrobial properties and is used to treat all kinds of infections, from those in the urinary tract to the symptoms of the common cold and flu. It is anti-inflammatory and its strong aromatic nature is good for clearing congested sinuses as well as using as a mouthwash. It has long been a common ingredient in many toothpastes.

If you are suffering from the first tickle of a sore throat that inevitably leads to a cold, then gargle with a strong infusion of thyme tea and honey. One of thyme's chief constituents is thymol, which has powerful antimicrobial properties and in vitro studies have shown it can inhibit the growth of both the yeast *Candida albicans* and the bacteria Staphylococcus. There is a growing interest in thyme's potential as a tool against antibiotic-resistant bacteria. It is also widely used in beekeeping to keep varroa mite at bay.

Thyme is also a powerful digestive and is traditionally combined with fatty meats, such as lamb and pork and even beef, to aid digestion.

In very large quantities thyme can be very beneficial against bloating, belching and farting. It can also help to calm digestive spasms and has a long history for being used as a vermifuge (to help the body get rid of parasites and worms). If you can't digest your supper for want of overindulging, then make a strong thyme tea and drink before bed.

# How to grow

Sunny, well-drained soil and regular picking are the keys to healthy thyme. Never let it sit somewhere damp over winter and feed it with liquid fertilizer in the summer if it looks a little wanting. If growing in a pot, make sure its roots have room to roam. It may be low-growing, but its roots like to spread shallowly across a pot. Low alpine terracotta pots are ideal as is a hanging basket. You should pick before the plant flowers for medicinal purposes, but for cooking the flowers are a nice addition.

Thyme is easiest dried on the stem and then rubbed off for storage. Shop-bought dried thyme is boring, but home-dried stuff has plenty of uses. If you buy fresh thyme from the shop and find you have more than you need, then spread it out on a baking tray to dry.

*Thymus vulgaris* 'English Broadleaf' has particularly wide leaves for cooking. Creeping thyme, *Thymus serpyllum*, is very low-growing with tiny leaves, woody stems and highly scented flowers.

# How to use

Start with 1 teaspoon of dried herbs or 1 tablespoon of fresh herbs in 250ml of boiling water, covered and steeped for 10 minutes up to three times a day. You can increase your daily allowance to up to 8g of dried herbs a day.

## Thyme oxymel

An oxymel is a very old herbal vinegar and is made by combining vinegar, herbs and honey (see page 115). Oxymels are delicious and an easy way to take herbs throughout the winter to ward off colds, flu and other respiratory symptoms.

Take 1 tablespoon an hour for a sore throat or congested cough.

You can take the oxymel straight or you can use it as a base for a salad dressing and you have your daily medicine and lunch sorted in one.

I make my oxymels with equal parts honey and vinegar and add a good handful of herbs. If you want a runnier version, you can use two parts vinegar.

2 handfuls fresh thyme                      Local, unpasteurized honey

Raw organic cider vinegar, preferably with the mother – the compound of bacteria and yeasts that ferments the cider and is left unfiltered in raw ciders. It is usually sold as 'vinegar with the mother' or 'unfiltered'.

Mince two good handfuls of fresh thyme and place in a large jar with the honey and vinegar. Cover the jar with a non-metallic lid; the vinegar will corrode the lid otherwise. If you have a metallic lid, use parchment paper between the metal and the liquid.

Shake the mixture once a day for 2 weeks. Strain out the mash and then store in the fridge. The oxymel will last for a year.

## Moth repellent

Thyme is an excellent moth repellent and can be used dried and placed between wool clothing, blankets, etc. If you're fussy about dried bits of thyme, then put it between layers of muslin.

# WATERCRESS

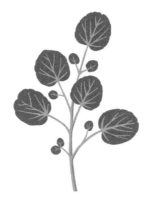

**Other Name** Yellowcress.

**Botanical Name** *Nasturtium officinale.*

**Family** Brassicaceae (cabbage family).

**Parts Used** Leaves, stems, flowers.

**Plant Properties** Nutritive, appetite-stimulant, diuretic, expectorant, laxative.

**Uses** Cleansing herb, high in vitamins and minerals.

**Preparations** Culinary.

**Considerations** None known.

I am not sure that anyone considers watercress a herb, but it's just too good to miss out on and a doddle to grow. Since we've been on the Earth we've been eating watercress. Along with cucumbers it can lay claim to being one of our oldest known vegetables. Over the centuries many claims have been made for its health benefits. When Hippocrates founded one of the first hospitals he grew watercress in the nearby natural springs to treat blood disorders. It's said that Captain James Cook was able to circumnavigate the globe three times in part due to his sailors' diet of watercress.

Recently, limited scientific studies have found that watercress consumed in quantities may protect cells from the damaging effect of free radicals and may also protect cells against DNA damage. The interesting thing about these studies is that people just ate watercress as a vegetable rather than it being a lab test on vegetable extracts. Now, the downside to all this is the sheer quantity of watercress you have to eat. Participants, who were all smokers, ate 85g of fresh watercress every day for eight weeks. But the jury is still out because you'd need a much larger, longer study to determine whether the effects of watercress on cells seen by the researchers actually translate into a decreased risk of cancer, but one thing is for sure: for a leafy vegetable it's packed with vitamins. It is particularly rich in vitamin K and contains significant amounts of vitamins A and C, riboflavin, vitamin B6, calcium and manganese. Watercress is a vitamin kick and a half, and you could be picking it daily from your back door.

## How to grow

As watercress is a semi-aquatic plant it will need to grow near water. It tends to do best in slightly alkaline conditions, hence its appearance in chalk streams, but it can be grown in normal garden compost. You'll need a bucket or an old tin bath. You could grow it in a pond, but if there's a risk of potential bacteria and contamination from groundwater running into the pond, then this isn't a good idea.

The seeds can be sown year-round; this is quickest indoors on a windowsill in a seed tray or small pot. Watercress makes excellent microgreens. Sow the seed liberally in a seed tray and harvest the leaves with scissors when they are just 5–8cm high. If you live in a flat with no outdoor space, this might be your best option. You can usually get two, perhaps three, cuts of baby leaves per tray.

If you do want to grow watercress outside, when the seedlings are large enough to handle carefully tease them apart and plant out in their final position in a container that is damp but not waterlogged. Once the seedlings start to grow, flood the container once or twice a week so that the watercress floats. The watercress doesn't want to sit in boggy conditions, so it's a good idea to have a few very small drainage holes in your container so that it drains very slowly. Don't overcrowd the seedlings; give them 10–15cm each way. Although watercress is perennial, I find it starts to lose its vigour after its second year. I let it flower and self-seed. It will happily find its own spot and after a wet spring I often find it sprouting in the garden.

If you can't find seed, you can propagate it with shop-bought watercress. In any given bag there will be a stem with tiny white roots appearing just below the leaf node. Sit these in water like you would cut flowers and watch those roots grow. Within days you will have 2.5cm long roots and you can plant these out. Take your cutting in early summer and plant out. Although watercress will root all year round, the shop-bought sort may have been grown undercover and might not like the rude awakening of winter outdoors.

Despite being hardy it will stop growing, so throw a little fleece over it to ensure you have a winter harvest.

# How to use

If you grow your watercress at home, give it a good wash, chop and eat as regularly as you like. Watercress is a laxative, so if you eat too much in one sitting you may find quick results. It is also incredibly peppery, which some people find too hard on their stomach. Watercress can be blanched, but never boil as you lose too many nutrients that way.

If you are lucky enough to find watercress growing in the wild, be incredibly cautious before you try it raw. It is very easy to get liver flukes from cattle and sheep on the watercress. This can cause fascioliasis, which is a very nasty disease that can result in liver failure. Watercress from the wild must be cooked, as heat kills the flukes.

# YARROW

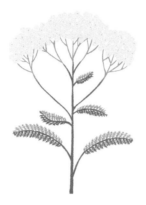

**Other Names** Common yarrow, staunchweed, soldier's woundwort, thousand-seal sanguinary, knights' milefoil, knyghten, carpenter's weed, bloodwort, devil's nettle, old man's pepper.

**Botanical Name** *Achillea millefolium.*

**Family** Asteraceae (sunflower or daisy family).

**Parts Used** Aerial parts, and the flowers or leaves and young stems harvested in the flowering stage, fresh or dried.

**Plant Properties** Reduces fever, hypotensive, astringent, anti-inflammatory, antispasmodic, diuretic, antimicrobial.

**Uses** Colds, flu, aids digestion, urinary tract infections, wound-healing, diarrhoea.

**Preparations** Culinary, infusions, poultices, teas.

**Considerations** Yarrow can cause skin inflammation and dermatitis in some people. This herb can be toxic to dogs, cats and horses, causing vomiting. It can also cause a rare severe allergic skin reaction that can increase the skin photosensitivity if overused as a medicine or when wet skin comes into contact with a combination of cut grass and yarrow.

**Not to be used during pregnancy.**

Yarrow is a wildflower often found in our summer meadows, but it is robust enough that it has moved itself into the more fertile, rank grasslands of parks, recreation grounds, roadsides and lawns. It's not hard, even in a city, to find a patch of yarrow growing merrily where the cutter blades can't catch it. It has flat, plate-like clusters of tiny white flowers and the leaves are feathery and distributed evenly along the stem, arranged spirally, more or less clasping. It has a strong, sweet scent much like chrysanthemum and is always visited by many pollinators. It is a food source for many insects and an important ecological plant for this reason.

It grows in many temperate regions of the northern hemisphere and has been introduced as livestock feed in many others. Its many common names indicate a long folkloric history: staunchweed, soldier's woundwort, thousand-seal sanguinary, knights' milefoil, knyghten, carpenter's weed, bloodwort, devil's nettle and old man's pepper. During the Roman period it was known as *herbal militaris* for its use in staunching the flow of blood from wounds. Its genus name, *Achillea*, is derived from the mythical Greek character Achilles, who reportedly carried the herb with him and his army to treat battle wounds.

It is a classic styptic and will stem bleeding, while its antiseptic properties treat infections. It's a brilliant herb for cuts and grazes. It is also a bitter tonic and if taken before eating will improve digestion. Hot yarrow tea will make you sweat, but can also reduce a fever and is said to aid restful sleep. It is also widely used in Native American herbal medicine. The Ojibwe sprinkle an infusion of the leaves on hot stones and inhale for headaches. The dried flowers are also placed on coals and the smoke inhaled to break a fever. The flowers were used in the Middle Ages to flavour beer prior to the introduction of hops.

# How to grow

There are numerous cultivars of yarrow for the garden, ranging from crimson to pale pink and yellows, although only the straight species, *A. millefolium*, is used medicinally. Yarrows like well-drained soil, but will tolerate damper conditions and full sun. They hate competition and often last just a few years in the garden before other, more robust perennials overtake them. If you want to plant this one, make sure it grows with plants that won't outstrip it. It can reach up to 1 metre tall, but usually grows to 50–60cm. You can sow seeds in spring; it requires temperatures of around 18–24°C/68–75°F and the seed needs light for germination, so don't bury it. To prolong its rather short life you can divide it in spring every other year, planting the divisions 30–45cm apart.

# How to use

### Yarrow tea
You can make a tea or infusion that can either be drunk to reduce a fever or used diluted to wash or bathe wounds. To make an infusion pour 250ml of boiling water over 1–2 teaspoons of dried herb, or 1–2 tablespoons of fresh herb, and infuse for 10–15 minutes, covered. This can be drunk hot three times a day.

### For medicinal use
A poultice of the fresh flowers or whole aerial parts can be made by bruising or mashing the leaves and it is said that it can even help with

deep cuts. It's brilliant for hikers, rock climbers and mountain bikers as it is nearly always found growing in open grassy places in mountains.

## Other species

English mace, *Achillea ageratum*, is an underrated herb that deserves more popularity. True mace, the outer husk of nutmeg, tastes of nutmeg, but also of cinnamon and coriander. English mace has definite hints of cinnamon but has clear notes of basil and ends on something very perfumed. If true mace tastes of nutmeg and spice, English mace tastes of a meadow. And perhaps that is why it is not so popular because if you were looking for something to add to apple pie, this is not it. It seems to go particularly well in potato salads, with chicken and white-fleshed fish, pork, cream soups and white sauces. It should be added at the end of cooking so that the perfumed notes don't turn bitter.

It's a lovely garden plant with many creamy-white tiny daisy flowers and strong stems that seem unyielding even to strong winds. It flowers from July right through to September, prefers full sun and can be grown in a variety of soils. In the medieval period it was used as a strewing herb for the floor to repel insects, lice and ticks and to make private rooms smell good.

# GLOSSARY

**Abortifacient** – a substance that induces abortion.

**Active constituent** – the active ingredient in a plant that has a medicinal effect on the body.

**Analgesic** – a painkilling medicine.

**Antifungal** – a substance that inhibits fungal infections.

**Antihistamine** – a substance that relieves symptoms of allergies, such as insect bites, hay fever, hives and itching.

**Anti-inflammatory** – a substance that reduces inflammation or swelling.

**Antimicrobial** – a substance that kills microorganisms or stops their growth.

**Antioxidant** – a substance that inhibits potentially damaging oxidizing agents in living organisms.

**Antispasmodic** – a substance that relieves involuntary spasms of muscles.

**Antiviral** – a substance that kills or inhibits viral infection.

**Aromatic** – an aromatic compound is an organic compound that has special stability and properties due to its closed loop of electrons. Perhaps more interestingly, aromatics in plants often smell pleasant and distinct.

**Astringent** – a substance that causes the contraction of skin cells and other tissues.

**Biennial** – a plant that flowers in its second year, sets seed and then dies. A foxglove is a good example.

**Carminative** – a substance that relieves farting and the bloating associated with it.

Compress – a soaked pad of absorbent material or a substance to relieve inflammation or stop bleeding.

Counterirritant – a substance that creates a very mild irritation or inflammation in one location to lessen the discomfort and/or inflammation in another location.

Decoction – a strong concentrated liquid extracted from a plant part, often the roots or bark, by boiling.

Decongestant – a substance to relieve a stuffy nose and congestion in the upper respiratory tract.

Demulcent – a substance relieving inflammation or irritation.

Diaphoretic – something that induces heavy sweating.

Diuretic – a substance that increases the production of urine.

Emmenagogue – a substance that stimulates or increases menstrual flow.

Emollient – something that softens and soothes skin.

Essential oil – a concentrated hydrophobic (water-repelling) liquid that contains volatile aromatic compounds. This means that they have a strong and distinct smell.

Expectorant – a substance that promotes and helps loosen the secretion of sputum in the air passages. It means a more productive cough.

Hepatotoxic – damaging or destructive to the liver.

Hypotensive – lowers the blood pressure.

Infusion – the process by which you extract chemical compounds from plant material in a solvent, such as water, oil, alcohol or vinegar.

Inulin – a carbohydrate that forms important dietary fibre which occurs naturally in many plants, particularly in the roots, rhizomes and tubers.

Lymphatic system – a system of tubes and lymph nodes that run through the body and which is an important part of our immune system.

Nervine – a substance used to calm the nerves.

Nutritive – a substance that provides nourishment.

Overwinter – to store a plant somewhere protected from frost, snow and winter weather.

Perennial – a plant that lives for more than two years.

Phytophototoxicity – often associated with phytophotodermatitis, which is skin burn or dermatitis caused after contact with light-sensitizing sap from a plant and then subsequent exposure to sunlight. Often found in the Euphorbiaceae and Rutaceae family.

Pinch out – pinching out is a kind of pruning, where the very top, soft growth of a plant is removed to encourage branching out below and to create a bushier habit.

Poultice – a soft, moist mass of material that is applied to a wound to relieve soreness, inflammation and infection. Poultices are often kept in place with a cloth.

Prebiotics – compounds in food, often forms of dietary fibre that help the growth or activity of beneficial microorganisms, such as bacteria and fungi in your gut microbiome.

Pricking out – a term used to describe removing seedlings once they have germinated in their own pot or module so they develop a strong root system.

Probiotics – live microorganisms in food such as yoghurt and fermented foods that improve or restore the gut microbiome.

Relaxant – a substance that promotes relaxation or reduces tension, such as a muscle relaxant.

Rhizome – a horizontal underground stem that sends out shoots and roots.

Runner – a stolon, which is a stem that grows just below or on the surface of the ground and forms a new plant.

Sedative – promoting or inducing a calm sleep.

Sepal – a part of a flower that encloses the petals and is typically green and leaf-like.

Strewing – to scatter or spread material.

Styptic – a substance that stems or stops bleeding when applied to a wound.

**Taproot** – a straight, tapered main root from which other roots sprout laterally. Think of a parsnip or carrot.

**Tonic** – in herbalism a tonic is a solution that helps to restore, tone and invigorate a system in the body.

**Topical** – a substance, usually a cream, that is applied directly to a part of the body.

**Vasodilatory** – widens the blood vessels.

**Vermifuge** – a substance that destroys or expels intestinal worms, such as tapeworms.

**Volatile oil** – *see* essential oil.

**Vulnerary** – a substance that heals a wound.

**Winnow** – to blow air through or over seeds to remove the chaff.

# A SHORT BIBLIOGRAPHY

Grieve, Maud and Leyel, C. F., *A Modern Herbal*. Jonathan Cape, 1931.
  Written in the 1930s, this remains a classic text for both foragers and herbalists, and is a joy to read. You'll often find this one at charity shops, so pick
  up a bargain and spend the rest of your life referring to it. Some information
  is dated, so cross-reference.

Hoffman, David, *Medical Herbalism: The Science and Practice of Herbal Medicine*. Healing Arts Press, 2003.
  An American text but hugely valuable in depth and a very comprehensive
  reference book that blends clinically orientated science with a holistic
  approach to herbal healing.

Chown, Vicky and Walker, Kim, *The Handmade Apothecary: Healing Herbal Remedies*. Kyle Books, 2017.
  Fantastic recipes for creams, tinctures, teas, balms and oils, and includes a very
  good chapter on foraging and a detailed A to Z of herbs.

De La Forêt, Rosalee, *The Alchemy of Herbs: Transform Everyday Ingredients into
  Foods and Remedies That Heal*. Hay House, 2017.
  An American text that looks at herbal medicine through cooking. Incredibly
  well-referenced text that marries a systematic, scientific approach to beautiful recipes that heal.

Cech, Richo, *Making Plant Medicine*. Herbal Reads, 2016.
  Probably the book I refer to most. Richo is a highly regarded US grower and
  nurseryman at Strictly Medicinal Seeds, and this book is an indispensable
  guide on how to use herbs at home. Along with *The Medicinal Herb Grower: A
  Guide for Cultivating Plants That Heal (Volume 1)*, these texts tell you everything

you need to know about home herbal growing, to say little of his wonderful seed list. https://strictlymedicinalseeds.com/

De Baïracli Levy, Juliette, *The Illustrated Herbal Handbook for Everyone*. Penguin, 1982.

De Baïracli Levy, Juliette, *Common Herbs for Natural Health*. Ash Tree Publishing, 1996.

I hold 'Juliette of the Herbs' dear to my heart because, more than anyone else, it was her work that led me to have a go, to experiment, to dabble and ultimately fall in love. It's also worth seeking out the documentary *Juliette of the Herbs*, which was made in 1998 about her life, her breeding of Afghan hounds and her travels around the world with many nomadic peoples from whom she learnt about herbal medicine.

# INDEX

These are herbs that will help with these common ailments. Please refer to the full entry in the book before using.

| | |
|---|---|
| Antibacterial | Basils, Dill, Eucalyptus, Fennel, Garlic, Horseradish, Lavender, Lemon balm, Marjoram, Myrtle, Perilla, Plantain, Rosemary, Selfheal, Sorrel, Thyme |
| Anti-dandruff | Nettle, Parsley, Rosemary |
| Antifungal infections | Calendula, Garlic, Lavender, Lemongrass, Rosemary, Selfheal, Thyme |
| Anti-inflammatory | Ashwagandha, Borage, Bugle, Calendula, Chickweed, Lady's mantle, Lime blossom, Mallows, Meadowsweet, Myrtle, Nettle, Perilla, Pines, Plantain, Raspberry, Rose, St John's wort, Sweet violet, Thistles |
| Anxiety | Camomile, Hawthorn, Hops, Lavender, Lemon Balm, Marjoram, Poppies, Rose, Rue |
| Aphrodisiac | Ashwagandha |
| Appetite-stimulant | Basils, Caraway, Dill, Marjoram, Sorrel |
| Bad breath | Dill, Fennel, Parsley |
| Bruises | Mallows, Selfheal, Sweet violet |
| Burns, sunburn | Aloe, Camomile, Marigold, St John's wort |
| Calms and relaxes nerves and organs | Feverfew, Hops, Lavender, Lime blossom, Oats |
| Chest infections | Elderflower, Horseradish |
| Chilblains | Chilli |
| Cleansing | Clevers, Garlic, Watercress |
| Colds | Chilli (to ward off), Elderberry (to ward off), Eucalyptus, Garlic, Horseradish, Hyssop, Lemon balm, Lime blossom, Marjoram, Nettle, Perilla, Pines, Rose, Savory, Thyme, Yarrow |

| Coughs | Angelicas (expectorant), Eucalyptus, Hyssop, Lemon balm, Lemongrass, Myrtle, Perilla, Pines, Sweet violet, Thyme |
|---|---|
| Cramps/colic | Borage, Camomile, Caraway, Coriander, Dill, Rue |
| Decongestant (temporary) | Mint |
| Digestive issues | Aloe, Angelicas, Artichokes, Basils, Camomile, Caraway, Chervil, Coriander, Dandelion, Dill, Fennel, Garlic, Hawthorn, Lady's mantle, Lemon balm, Lemongrass, Lovage, Marjoram, Mint, Myrtle, Parsley, Raspberry, Rose, Rosemary, Savory, Tarragon, Thyme, Yarrow |
| Drawing poultice | Bugle, Plantain |
| Energy-building | Ashwagandha |
| Exhaustion | Oats |
| Eye wash | Camomile, Chervil |
| Flatulence | Basils, Caraway, Dill, Fennel, Lovage, Myrtle, Savory, Tarragon, Thyme |
| Flu | Camomile, Chilli, Elderflower, Garlic, Lime Blossom, Rose, Tarragon, Yarrow |
| Gas/bloating | Dill, Savory, Tarragon |
| Gastritis | Meadowsweet |
| Hayfever | Elderflower, Nettle |
| Headaches | Lavender, Poppies, Rue |
| Heartburn | Caraway, Dill, Fennel, Meadowsweet |
| Improves circulation | Chilli, Hawthorn, Pines, Rosemary, Savory |
| Insect bites | Bugle, Lavender, Lemongrass, Lemon balm, Mallows, Plantain, Savory |
| Insomnia/aids sleep/sedative | Camomile, Hops, Lavender, Lemongrass, Lime blossom, Poppies, Tarragon |
| Liver tonic | Artichokes, Dandelion, Thistles |
| Mastitis | Lady's mantle |
| Menstrual problems | Borage, Caraway, Lady's mantle, Rosemary |
| Migraines | Camomile, Feverfew, Lime blossom |
| Mild anaesthetic for nerve/muscle pain e.g. toothache | Chilli, St John's wort |
| Mild diuretic | Borage, Dandelion |
| Motion sickness | Camomile |
| Mouth ulcers | Lady's mantle (as a gargle), Lemon balm, Selfheal |
| Nausea | Hyssop, Marjoram, Meadowsweet |
| Nervousness | Lemon balm |
| Oral health: gingivitis, gum health, mouth ulcers | Lady's mantle (as a gargle), Lemon balm, Myrtle (as a gargle), Sage, Selfheal |
| Parasites | Garlic |
| Piles | Dill |

| | |
|---|---|
| Poor circulation | Chilli, Garlic, Hawthorn |
| Poultice for skin inflammation | Chickweed, Cleavers |
| Rashes | Camomile |
| Reduces fever | Sorrel, Tarragon |
| Reduces inflammation in body | Borage |
| Relaxant | Lime blossom |
| Respiratory conditions | Mallows, Sweet violet (upper respiratory infections), Thyme |
| Scalp tonic | Sage |
| Sedative | Ashwagandha, Hops, Mint, Thyme |
| Sinusitis | Myrtle |
| Skin issues | Calendula, Camomile, Chickweed, Lemongrass, Oats, Plantain, Rose, Sweet violet |
| Sleeplessness | Oats, Poppies |
| Soothes the gut/ digestive tract | Marigold, Rosemary |
| Sore throat | Raspberry, Rose, Rosemary, Sage, Selfheal, Thyme |
| Sprains | St John's wort |
| Spring tonic | Chervil, Cleavers (to stimulate lymphatic system), Nettle, Plantain |
| Stimulates hair follicles and increases circulation to the scalp | Rosemary |
| Stimulates immune system | Elderberry, Horseradish, Hyssop |
| Stomach cramps | Marjoram |
| Strengthens and tones the uterus before going into labour | Raspberry |
| Stress | Lemon balm, Oats |
| Sweetens and increases breast milk supply | Fennel |
| Teething | Camomile |
| Tension pains | Mint |
| Toothache | Chilli, Tarragon |
| Urinary tract infections | Angelicas (antiseptic), Yarrow |
| Viral infections | Elderflower, Lemon balm |
| Vitamin and mineral boost | Sorrel, Watercress |
| Wounds/cuts/ulcers/ insect bites/boils | Bugle, Chervil, Chickweed, Eucalyptus, Lady's mantle (as a styptic), Lavender, Lemongrass, Lemon balm, Mallows, Marigold, Marjoram, Parsley, Perilla, Plantain, Savory, Selfheal, St John's wort, Yarrow |

# ACKNOWLEDGEMENTS

To Barbara Wilkinson, whose passion for herbs is infectious, thank you for your guidance, support and enthusiasm for this project. Thanks also to the Herb Society of Great Britain for introducing me to such a warm and wonderful world of herb lovers; to Tom Frost for his brilliant illustrations; to Fenella, Zennor and the rest of the team at Penguin; to the wonderful Jennie Roman for her thoughtful and meticulous edit of this book; to my agent, Cath Summerhayes; to everyone who has sipped my teas and tried my potions; and particularly to Ming De Nasty and Sara Wilson for their love and support. Thank you to my mum and dad for teaching me, each in their own way, that plants are powerful medicines. Finally, to the wonderful Ele, this book is dedicated to you. May there be many herbs in your future life as a doctor.